D1567383

Cancer, HIV and AIDS

CANCER SURVEYS

Advances and Prospects in Clinical, Epidemiological and Laboratory Oncology

Published for the

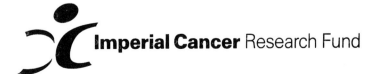

Imperial Cancer Research Fund

Cancer, HIV and AIDS

Guest Editors
V Beral
H W Jaffe
R A Weiss

COLD SPRING HARBOR LABORATORY PRESS 1991

CANCER SURVEYS
Cancer, HIV and AIDS
Volume 10

Copyright 1991 by Imperial Cancer Research Fund
Published by Cold Spring Harbor Laboratory Press
Printed in the United States of America
ISBN 0-87969-362-2
ISSN 1050-849X

Cover and book design by Leon Bolognese & Associates, Inc.

All Cold Spring Harbor Laboratory Press publications may be ordered directly from Cold Spring Harbor Laboratory Press, 10 Skyline Drive, Plainview, New York 11803-9729. Phone: Continental US & Canada 1–800–843–4388; all other locations (516) 349–1930. FAX: (516) 349–1946.

Contents

Preface

When I first became involved in medicine and later in cancer research, over 50 years ago, it was still just possible for an educated physician or cancer scientist to comprehend at least the basic concepts and significance of work in progress. Forty years later this was no longer possible. *Cancer Surveys* was first published in 1982 as a modest attempt to approach this problem. It also marked a new departure for the Imperial Cancer Research Fund. Although many of the basic concepts in experimental cancer research, including the classic "Draft Scheme for Enquiring into the Nature, Cause, Prevention and Treatment of Cancer" by E. F. Bashford,* the Fund's first director, appeared in the *Annual Reports* published by the Fund, our publishing activities were restricted in the main to descriptions of work carried out in the Fund's own laboratories.

Cancer Surveys had a wider scope and offered a comprehensive review of aspects of oncology that were currently interesting. A major objective was to bridge the gap between the clinic, the laboratory and the epidemiologist in the field. Each issue featured a single topic and was intended to provide a critical account of the current state of knowledge, major problems and possible ways forward, written by leaders in the field. Looking back over nearly 10 years of issues, I believe *Cancer Surveys* has successfully achieved those goals.

For its second decade it is particularly appropriate that *Cancer Surveys* is to be published for us by Cold Spring Harbor Laboratory, an institute like our own, founded about the same time and with which we have many scientific and personal contacts. In addition, the publishing traditions of its press complement those of *Cancer Surveys.* The layout and format of the new series have been improved and by using electronic publishing techniques we have been able to reduce delays in publication even further. My own thanks are due to Christine Sinclair at Imperial Cancer Research Fund and Nancy Ford, Mary Cozza, Leon Bolognese and John Inglis at Cold Spring Harbor Laboratory Press for their efforts in planning and production.

Cancer Surveys is available on subscription or as single issues and is published as a service to all concerned with tumour biology, research and the care of patients with cancer. Its specific aims are detailed in our Policy Statement printed on the back cover. Although inevitably there is an emphasis in some issues on cell and molecular biology and genetics, a glance at the contents of earlier volumes and those now in

---

*Third Scientific Report of the Imperial Cancer Research Fund 1908 reprinted in full in the Journal of the National Cancer Institute (*19*, 307 [1957]) on the 20th anniversary of the establishment of the National Cancer Institute, Bethesda, Maryland USA.

preparation shows that each attempts a synthesis of current knowledge in the topics covered and their possible clinical applications.

My preface to the first issue of *Cancer Surveys* concluded with the following comments:

> With many journals publishing reports directly related to cancer and innumerable others dealing with the enormous range of biological topics which are of interest to cancer workers, yet another journal would seem to be superfluous. Paradoxically this vast output makes this publication of even greater importance and we hope that it will perform as useful (although different) a purpose as the original reports published by the Imperial Cancer Research Fund.

> In its new form, in association with Cold Spring Harbor Laboratory Press, *Cancer Surveys* should be able to achieve its purpose with even more success.

L M FRANKS, MD

Cancer, HIV and AIDS

Overview: Cancer, HIV and AIDS

VALERIE BERAL • HAROLD JAFFE • ROBIN WEISS

One in six people with acquired immunodeficiency syndrome (AIDS) in the USA or Europe also have cancer, albeit unusual cancers such as Kaposi's sarcoma or non-Hodgkin lymphoma. This volume summarizes current knowledge of the causes of cancer in people with AIDS, the epidemiology of these cancers and their clinical manifestations and treatment. Emphasis is on Kaposi's sarcoma and on non-Hodgkin lymphoma, since the risk of these two malignancies is substantially increased by human immunodeficiency virus (HIV) infection. The list of other cancers whose risk might also be increased by HIV infection is long (see Rabkin and Blattner, this issue), but for none, except perhaps Hodgkin's disease, is there more than anecdotal evidence of an association.

Before the AIDS epidemic, Kaposi's sarcoma in the USA and Europe was a rare, relatively benign condition of elderly men. Its unusual appearance in young and middle aged homosexual men in New York and California heralded the AIDS epidemic. Although the pathology of the lesions in HIV infected individuals was similar to that in HIV uninfected individuals, the clinical manifestations were so different that AIDS related Kaposi's sarcoma was initially thought to be a distinct condition, with an entirely different cause from other forms of Kaposi's sarcoma. There is now a growing consensus that Kaposi's sarcoma is caused by an as yet unidentified transmissible agent and that the same agent causes all forms of Kaposi's sarcoma. Indeed, some have gone so far as to suggest that Kaposi's sarcoma is not even a true malignancy. It now seems likely that there are symptom free carriers of the Kaposi's agent and that an individual's immune status determines the clinical manifestations of disease—the more intense the immunosuppression, the more disseminated and rapidly growing are the Kaposi's lesions and the more aggressive is the disease.

The epidemiological pattern of Kaposi's sarcoma in patients with AIDS provides tantalizing clues to the mode of transmission of the agent that causes Kaposi's sarcoma. The very high risk of Kaposi's sarcoma among homosexual men with AIDS, with around one in five affected, suggests that sexual transmission is likely to be common. Since oral-anal contact may be part of the sexual activity of homosexual men, these findings are also consistent with faecal-oral spread of the agent. Transmission via blood, blood products and perinatally probably occurs as well but to a lesser extent than sexual transmission, since only 1 in 30 or fewer AIDS subjects who acquired the HIV parenterally or perinatally also has Kaposi's sarcoma. The epidemiological evidence further suggests that the agent was not prevalent in northern Europe or the USA until recently and that it was relatively common in parts of central and eastern Africa, the Caribbean and the Mediterranean before then. Efforts are now underway to identify the specific causal agent, perhaps a new retrovirus, mycoplasma, enterovirus or other virus. With the current speed of laboratory research the agent might be identified soon.

Non-Hodgkin lymphoma affects about 1 in 30 people with AIDS in the USA or Europe. There is little doubt that the histological types of the lymphomas that occur in association with HIV infection are atypical. The large majority of the lymphomas are high grade malignancies, and Burkitt's lymphoma is not uncommon. As yet there is no consensus on how to classify these lymphomas, and in the meantime some researchers have devised their own system, as is described in Herndier (this issue). There is an obvious need for standard definitions and nomenclature here. The clinical manifestations of the lymphomas in people with AIDS are unusual as well. Extranodal involvement is common, and primary lesions of the brain are highly characteristic of an association with HIV infection. Response to therapy is disappointing.

It is widely believed that infectious agents may also be responsible for the AIDS associated lymphomas. As with Kaposi's sarcoma the immunosuppression associated with HIV infection probably results in clinical disease appearing in otherwise symptom free carriers. As yet there are few clues to the mode of transmission of the agent or agents that cause non-Hodgkin lymphoma in immunosuppressed people. The agents are probably not transmitted sexually or by blood or blood products, since the risk of developing a lymphoma is similar in those who acquired the HIV by homosexual or heterosexual activity or parenterally. The epidemiological evidence suggests that the same aetiological agent may cause certain lymphomas regardless of whether they are associated with HIV infection. The Epstein-Barr virus may well be involved in the pathogenesis of some of the lymphomas, but the evidence is conflicting. The role of other viruses, including human T lymphotropic virus (HTLV)-I, is currently being investigated.

It is probably not a coincidence that the two cancers that have been most strongly linked to HIV infection are both thought to have an infectious cause. The main conclusion to emerge from research into cancers associated with immunosuppressive therapy is that the cancers that appeared are the ones known to have or suspected of having an infectious cause, as reviewed in an earlier issue of *Cancer Surveys* (Vol 1, No 4; Penn, 1982). Relatively few patients have been treated with immunosuppressive therapy compared with the large numbers who are infected with HIV. Thus the AIDS epidemic is providing a natural experiment on a massive scale from which much can be learned about the role of immunosuppression in the development of cancer. In general, the cancers associated with HIV infection are similar to those associated with immunosuppressive therapy. But there are fascinating differences as well. Perhaps the most curious is that Burkitt's lymphoma is commonly associated with

HIV infection but rarely if at all with immunosuppressive therapy. Unravelling the reasons for this discrepancy may well enhance our understanding of the role of the immune system in the development and control of cancer.

Another challenge to researchers is to explain why Kaposi's sarcoma and Burkitt's lymphoma, which are both common in patients with HIV infection, were both endemic in certain parts of Africa—eastern Zaire and Uganda—before the AIDS epidemic. Clearly it is possible that the aetiological agents for these two cancers happened to be especially common in those areas, but what is particularly perplexing is that HIV is now believed to have originated from that very same part of Africa. The endemic form of Kaposi's sarcoma which was present in these areas before the AIDS epidemic has been shown to be not associated with HIV infection. As yet no adequate explanation exists for this unusual aggregation of such rare disorders.

With the spread of the HIV and the pace of modern research we can expect many questions raised in this volume to be answered soon. For example, we should soon know whether the risk of other cancers known or suspected to be caused by infectious agents—Hodgkin's disease, hepatocellular cancer and cervical cancer—are also increased in association with HIV infection. Research workers may also have identified the specific agents that cause Kaposi's sarcoma and certain forms of non-Hodgkin lymphoma. This should aid our understanding of the causes of cancer not only in the HIV infected but also in the HIV uninfected. As disastrous as the spread of HIV is, the insights that the AIDS epidemic provides into the causes of cancer may ultimately lead to new and successful approaches to cancer prevention.

Epidemiology of Kaposi's Sarcoma

VALERIE BERAL

ICRF Cancer Epidemiology Unit, Radcliffe Infirmary, Oxford OX2 6HE

INTRODUCTION

Why was an outbreak of Kaposi's sarcoma (KS) in homosexual men the first sign of the looming AIDS epidemic in the USA? Until the advent of AIDS, KS was exceedingly rare in the USA and Europe and was regarded as a relatively benign disorder of elderly men (Dörffel, 1932; Hansson, 1940; Ronchese and Kern, 1953; Oettle, 1962). It was known that the risk of KS was increased in immunosuppressed transplant recipients, but this was an unusual complication (Kinlen, 1982). Kaposi's sarcoma is about 300 times as common in HIV infected individuals as in other immunosuppressed groups, and it is 20 000 times as common as in the general population (Beral *et al*, 1990).

Another extraordinary feature of KS in people with AIDS is the extent to which its occurrence varies from one HIV transmission group to another. Most notable are the extremely high risks among homosexual and bisexual men (Table 1). In the USA and Europe, at least one in five homosexual men with AIDS also has KS. In contrast, only 1 in 30 or fewer intravenous drug users, haemophiliacs and transfusion recipients with AIDS also have KS. Moreover, as will be discussed later, an individual's risk for the development of KS is not constant within each HIV transmission group but has declined sharply over time and varies substantially according to where the individual lives and was born.

In this chapter, I describe the factors that determine KS risk in people with AIDS and discuss how this information provides clues to the aetiology of the disease. As Peterman and his colleagues argue elsewhere in this issue, the evidence points strongly to a transmissible agent, in addition to the HIV, as a cause of KS. The same transmissible agent may well cause all forms of KS whether or not the disease is associated with HIV infection. I therefore begin with a brief description of the so-called "endemic" and "classical" forms of KS, which occur in the absence of HIV infection.

KAPOSI'S SARCOMA IN HIV UNINFECTED PEOPLE

Kaposi's sarcoma in HIV uninfected individuals is so rare that less is known about it than about the same condition in HIV infected individuals. The three most prominent features of KS in HIV uninfected people are its strong predilection for men, its benign clinical course and the striking geographical variability in its incidence, with pockets of high incidence in central and eastern Africa.

TABLE 1. Subjects with AIDS in various countries who were also reported to have Kaposi's sarcoma, by HIV transmission group

HIV transmission group	Percent of AIDS subjects who have Kaposi's sarcoma (reported no. of subjects with AIDS)		
	USA[a] (90 990)	UK[b] (2830)	Spain[c] (1074)
Homosexual or bisexual men	21%	23%	36%
Heterosexuals	3%	10%	0%
Intravenous drug users	2%	0%	2%
Transfusion recipients	3%	0%	0%
Haemophiliacs	1%	0%	0%
Children infected by perinatal transmission	1%	0%	0%

[a]Beral et al, 1990
[b]Beral et al, 1991
[c]Casabona et al, 1990

Kaposi's Sarcoma in Africa

Kaposi's sarcoma was relatively common in certain parts of Africa long before the striking spread of HIV, accounting for as many as 10% of all malignancies seen in some hospitals (Oettle, 1962; Hutt, 1984). During the 1960s and 1970s, its geographical distribution within Africa was distinctive. The disease was exceedingly rare in western and southern Africa and most common in central and eastern Africa, especially in Rwanda and Burundi and near the Zaire/Uganda border. This form of "endemic" KS was ten or more times as common in men as in women, and its incidence generally increased with age (Taylor *et al*, 1972). The disease was rare in children except before the age of 5 years.

The endemic form of KS in Africa is not associated with HIV infection and can be distinguished clinically from HIV associated disease by its relatively benign course and by the localized anatomical distribution of lesions (Bayley, this issue). The lesions of endemic KS are usually confined to the lower limbs and tend to develop slowly, whereas the lesions of HIV associated disease in Africans are disseminated throughout the body and tend to progress rapidly.

Clustering of KS in households has been described, and it has long been thought that the disease might be caused by an infectious agent (Oettle, 1962). Giraldo *et al* (1972) observed herpes like particles in KS lesions from African patients and proposed that the cytomegalovirus might be a cause of KS. Current evidence suggests that the cytomegalovirus is not the causal agent (Peterman *et al*, this issue).

Kaposi's Sarcoma in Europe and the USA

Kaposi's sarcoma was extremely rare in the West before the advent of AIDS (Dörffel, 1932; Hannson, 1940; Ronchese and Kern, 1953). As in Africa, males were predominantly affected, and there is considerable circumstantial evidence, mostly from case reports, that the incidence varied markedly from one country to another. The incidence seems to have been especially high in men from eastern Europe, Italy and other Mediterranean countries (Dörffel, 1932; Oettle, 1962). This form of "classical" KS generally occurred in old men and was rarely fatal. As with endemic African KS, lesions tended to be confined to the limbs and to progress slowly.

It has recently become clear that KS occurs in HIV uninfected as well as in HIV infected homosexual men. Following the first report of KS in six homosexual men from New York who were HIV negative (Friedman-Kien *et al*, 1990) there have been reports of KS in HIV negative homosexual men from many parts of the world (Kitchen *et al*, 1990; Muret *et al*, 1990). The clinical manifestations of the disease in these HIV negative homosexual men are similar to those described for classical KS, with lesions localized to the limbs and a benign course of the illness. Most cases reported were diagnosed in the late 1970s and 1980s, suggesting that there may be a small epidemic of KS in HIV negative homosexual men accompanying the massive epidemic of the disease in HIV positive homosexual men. Whether KS was especially common in homosexual men before the advent of AIDS is unknown, but the marked excess of both endemic and classical KS in males raises this possibility.

Sparse as the information is, there is some evidence that the severity of KS and the ages of those affected have changed in Europe during the past century. More than a century ago Moritz Kaposi (1872), a dermatologist working in Vienna, first described the disease in six men, half of whom were under 50 years of age. He commented that the disease was usually fatal in 2 to 3 years. Ten years later, in 1882, de Amici, a dermatologist working in Naples, described 11 men and 1 woman with a similar disease (translated by Ronchese, 1958). Six of the 12 whom de Amici described were under the age of 50, and he too commented that the disease was often rapidly fatal. By the 20th century case reports tended to be of considerably older men, most of whom had benign disease (Dörffel, 1932; Hannson, 1940; Ronchese and Kern, 1953). It is, of course, difficult to draw firm conclusions from case reports, but with the recent experience of an epidemic of an aggressive form of KS associated with HIV infection in middle aged men, the case reports of a century ago raise the possibility that a similar form of the disease might have existed before. Whether this was associated with immunosuppression can only be the subject of speculation. These intriguing anecdotes argue for further study of KS in HIV negative individuals.

The incidence of KS is reported to have doubled in Scandinavia during the 1970s (Bendsöe et al, 1990). A survey of the cases diagnosed in Sweden before the AIDS epidemic began indicated that previous blood transfusion or corticosteroid use may increase the risk of disease (Bendsöe et al, 1990). It was suggested that the agent causing KS might be transmitted by blood transfusion and that the immunosuppression associated with steroid use might increase susceptibility to the disease; the increasing use of these therapies may have contributed to the increased incidence of the disease in Sweden.

Association with Immunosuppression

Immunosuppressed subjects are at increased risk for the development of KS (Kinlen, 1982). The risk varies according to the country of origin of the patients—most of those in whom KS was reported to have developed after immunosuppressive treatment came from Africa, the Mediterranean or the Middle East (Penn, 1988). In Saudi Arabia, for example, KS is the most common tumour occurring after transplantation (Qunibi et al, 1988), whereas it rarely occurs in subjects from Britain, Australasia or the USA and is far less common than transplant associated lymphomas (Kinlen, 1982; Penn, 1988). Unlike endemic or classical KS, there is no marked excess of transplant associated KS in males.

The clinical manifestations of KS in the immunosuppressed are similar to those in HIV associated KS. Lesions are not confined to the limbs but are widely disseminated, frequently in the oral cavity and gastrointestinal tract.

Lesions tend to occur soon after transplantation, and the disease process has been reported to be halted and even reversed by the withdrawal of immunosuppressive drugs (Penn, 1988). This suggests that there may well be symptom free carriers of the causal agent and that immunosuppression results in clinical expression of the disease in carriers. Thus an individual's immunological status probably determines whether KS is expressed clinically and also the severity of the disease and the anatomical distribution of the associated lesions.

KAPOSI'S SARCOMA IN HIV INFECTED HOMOSEXUAL AND BISEXUAL MEN

HIV infection substantially increases KS risk, and homosexual and bisexual men with AIDS are far more likely to have KS than are others with AIDS (Table 1). The immunosuppression associated with HIV infection accounts in part for the increased risk, and it is likely that the immunosuppression results in aggressive clinical disease in people who would otherwise be symptom free carriers of the causal agent. But this does not explain the very high risks in homosexual men. The additional factor in homosexual men is likely to be that the KS causal agent, like HIV, is transmitted sexually. The risk of KS in affected homosexual and bisexual men is changing over time and varies considerably within a country according to where the men live, their sexual practices and the characteristics of their sexual partners. Kaposi's sarcoma is commonly the presenting symptom in homosexual men with AIDS (Lifson *et al*, 1990), and its characteristic clinical features in adults (Buchbinder and Friedman-Kien, this issue) are such that misdiagnosis is not a major problem for epidemiological studies.

Geographical Distribution

In the USA and the UK, homosexual and bisexual men with AIDS are most likely to have KS if they live in foci of the AIDS epidemic. In the USA for example, 30% of white homosexual and bisexual men with AIDS from California and New York were reported to have KS compared with only 5% of white homosexual and bisexual men with AIDS from Kansas (Fig. 1). No other reported complication of HIV infection has a similar geographical distribution within the USA. In the UK, homosexual and bisexual men from London are twice as likely to have KS reported as are men from other areas (Beral *et al*, 1991).

Association with Sexual Practices

Men with AIDS who are exclusively homosexual are twice as likely as bisexual men with AIDS to have KS (Peterman T, personal communication). This is

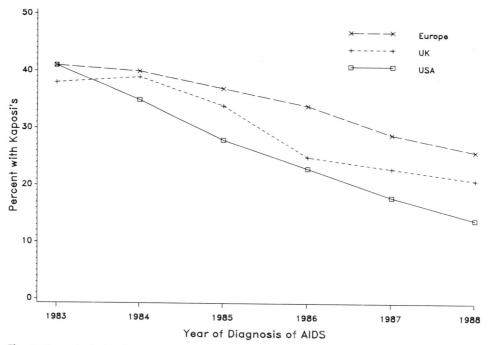

Fig. 1. Percent of white homosexual men with AIDS reported to have KS, by state in the USA (From Beral *et al*, 1990)

one of many sexual practices among men with AIDS that differ according to whether or not they have KS.

Six studies have contrasted the sexual practices of homosexual and bisexual men with KS with those of men with opportunistic infections or other manifestations of AIDS (Haverkos *et al*, 1985; Goedert, 1987; Moss *et al*, 1987; Archibald *et al*, 1990; Jacobsen *et al*, 1990; Lifson *et al*, 1990). All but the two early reports (Haverkos *et al*, 1985; Moss *et al*, 1987) were based on the follow-up of previously healthy men, and so information on sexual practices was obtained before AIDS developed in the men. As discussed below, clear differences in sexual practices were generally found between men with KS and those with other manifestations of AIDS. The men in whom KS developed tended to be more sexually active and to have had more past sexually transmitted infections than the men with other manifestations of AIDS, and they were more likely to have sexual partners who came from areas where KS is common. In addition, some results suggest that the men with KS were more likely than the other men to perform various sexual practices that involve contact with faeces.

Only one study, by Lifson *et al* (1990), did not find consistent differences. Their study population lived in San Francisco, and the information on sexual practices used in their analyses was the average of that reported between October 1983 and September 1986 (Lifson *et al*, 1990). Sexual behaviour is known to have changed markedly in San Francisco during that period (Darrow *et al*, 1987). If past practices and exposures determine an individual's risk of KS, then information on sexual practices at a time of rapid behaviour change may well not be relevant.

Table 2 summarizes the information available on the number of sexual partners of homosexual and bisexual men with AIDS according to whether or not they had KS. The way in which the number of sexual partners has been reported varies from one study to another, but in each study the men with KS tended to have the most sexual partners.

The type of sexual partner and sexual practices performed are probably more closely related to risk than is the number of partners. Homosexual men with AIDS who had KS are more likely to be sexual contacts of other men with KS (Auerbach *et al*, 1984). In addition, men with KS are more likely than men without KS to have met their partners in bathhouses and other places where casual anonymous sex is usual (Haverkos *et al*, 1985; Moss *et al*, 1987; Archibald *et al*, 1990).

Homosexual and bisexual men with KS are also more likely than men with other manifestations of AIDS to have sexual partners from localities where KS is known to be especially common. For example, homosexual and bisexual men with KS from Vancouver, Canada, were three times more likely to have sexual

TABLE 2. Reported number of male sexual partners of homosexual men with AIDS, according to whether or not the men had Kaposi's sarcoma

Measure of number of male sexual partners	Clinical manifestation of AIDS			
	Kaposi's sarcoma (no.)		Other opportunistic infection (no.)	
Percent with more than 100 sexual partners in the year before illness (Haverkos *et al*, 1985)	60%	(67)	30%[a]	(20)
Percent with more than 20 sexual partners per year (Moss *et al*, 1987)	81%	(108)	70%	(51)
Percent with more than 100 sexual partners in the past year (Goedert *et al*, 1987)	38%	(8)	30%	(10)
Percent with more than 20 sexual partners per year (Archibald *et al*, 1990)	76%	(25)	50%[a]	(57)
Median number of sexual partners in 1983–1986 (Lifson *et al*, 1990)				
steady	10	(71)	10	(109)
non-steady	285		243	

[a]Statistically significant difference between men with Kaposi's sarcoma and those with other manifestations of AIDS (p<0.05)

partners from California and New York than were men with other manifestations of AIDS (Archibald *et al*, 1990); and in the UK, homosexual and bisexual men with KS were twice as likely to have sexual partners from the USA as were men with other manifestations of AIDS (Beral *et al*, 1991).

There is some evidence that contact with faecal material, either by rimming (active oral-anal contact) or by fisting (insertion of the subject's hand into the partner's rectum) are important risk factors for KS. Moss and colleagues (1987) found a threefold increase in risk of KS associated with rimming (reported by Abrams, 1990). Jacobsen *et al* (1990) also found that rimming was more common in those with KS than in those with other manifestations of AIDS, but the difference was not statistically significant. Archibald *et al* (1990) noted a statistically significant doubling of risk associated with fisting but not with rimming. Goedert *et al* (1987) reported an increased risk of KS associated with frequent receptive oral-genital contact but not with oral-anal contact.

Most investigators have reported statistically significant associations of KS with a variety of past sexually transmitted infections, although the specific type of infection varied from one report to another and there was little consistency (Goedert *et al*, 1987; Moss *et al*, 1987; Abrams, 1990; Archibald *et al*, 1990; Jacobsen *et al*, 1990). Abrams (1990) argues that intestinal infections and the "gay bowel syndrome" were especially common in men with KS. It is difficult to evaluate the published information on past intestinal infections, since the results have not been systematically reported, but the findings reported by Goedert *et al* (1987) and Moss *et al* (1987, quoted by Abrams, 1990) would support Abrams' view.

The extremely high risk of KS in homosexual men and their frequent use of poppers (amyl or butyl nitrite inhalants) as sexual stimulants led Haverkos *et al* (1985) to suggest that the poppers themselves might be the cause of KS. The findings from subsequent studies have not supported that view (Goedert *et al*, 1987; Polk *et al*, 1987; Jacobsen *et al*, 1990; Lifson *et al*, 1990). Only Archibald *et al* (1990) found a significant association between popper use and KS risk after simultaneous adjustment for various sexual practices.

The types of sexual behaviour that have been associated with KS are highly correlated. Men with many sexual partners are especially likely to meet them in bathhouses and other public places, to use poppers and practice rimming and fisting and to have had various sexually transmitted infections in the past (Jaffe *et al*, 1983; Beral V, unpublished data).

Some authors have attempted to identify the most important exposures and behaviours for KS by statistical modelling of several risk factors simultaneously, and their conclusions have been varied (Haverkos *et al*, 1985; Goedert *et al*, 1987; Archibald *et al*, 1990). Vandenbroucke and Pardoel (1989) have illustrated the dangers of relying too heavily on statistical modelling in similar circumstances. Their review of the results of analyses aimed at uncovering the main risk factors for the development of AIDS before HIV was identified concluded that simultaneous statistical adjustment for various exposures and behaviours tended to point to false clues. In particular, they noted that several investigators mistakenly identified poppers as a more important risk factor for AIDS than sexual practices on the basis of statistical modelling. This erroneous conclusion was presumably because the main determinant of the risk of developing AIDS—sexual contact with an HIV infected partner—could not be assessed at that time, and popper use served as a better surrogate for it than did other measures. Similar problems exist when attempting to identify the main risk factors for KS in homosexual and bisexual men with AIDS.

There is little doubt that some aspect of sexual behaviour among highly sexually active men is the main determinant of KS risk in HIV infected homosexual men, and this suggests that the causal agent is transmitted sexually. But whether it is the number of sexual partners or some particular type of behaviour such as rimming that is important is still unclear. It is important to sort out which factors determine risk, since this would provide clues to the mode of transmission of the agent and thus the type of agent involved.

Time Trends

In the USA, the UK and Europe, the proportion of homosexual and bisexual men with AIDS who have KS has declined steadily over time (Fig. 2). The pro-

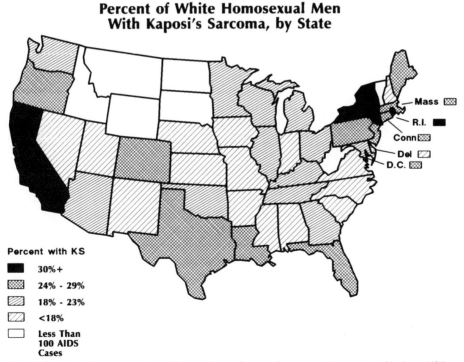

Fig. 2. Percent of homosexual and bisexual men from various countries reported to have KS by year of diagnosis of AIDS. Data for Europe from Casabona *et al* (1991); for the UK from Beral *et al* (1991); and for the USA from Beral *et al* (1990)

portion with KS approximately halved in the 5 years from 1983 to 1988. This decline is not due to changes in the definition of AIDS or to reporting biases but reflects a true substantial reduction in the proportion of homosexual and bisexual men with AIDS who have KS. Within the USA the relative decline has been most striking in young men and in whites (Beral *et al*, 1990). The decline would also seem to be more rapid in the USA than in the UK or Europe (Fig. 2).

The reasons for the decline are not entirely clear, although they are probably related to sexual practices. Perhaps the most important reason is that the homosexual or bisexual men who developed AIDS at the beginning of the epidemic were among the most sexually active, and these men were also the most likely to have KS. As the AIDS epidemic spread to less sexually active homosexual men, who are at lower risk of KS, so the proportion with KS has declined. Changing sexual behaviour and the reduction in the incidence of sexually transmitted diseases among homosexual men may also be playing a part.

Association with Age, Race and Genetic Markers

The risk of KS in homosexual men with AIDS varies little with age (Fig. 3). The typical finding for classical KS (an increasing risk with age) is not evident in men with AIDS—indeed, the reverse is found, the risk being lowest of all in

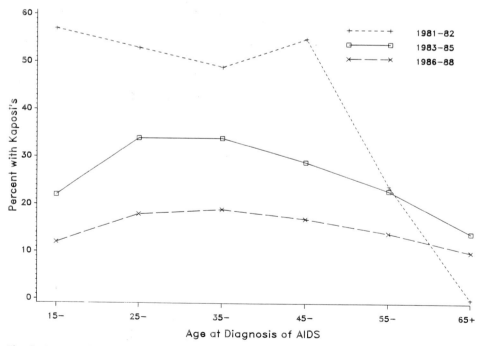

Fig. 3. Percent of homosexual and bisexual men with AIDS reported to have KS in the USA, by age and calendar year of diagnosis of AIDS (From Beral *et al*, 1990)

men with AIDS who are over 55 years of age. The age pattern has changed somewhat over time in the USA, with young men showing a greater proportionate decline in risk of KS than older men (Fig. 3). Some of the recent generation of young men would not have become sexually active until after the AIDS epidemic began, and their relatively low risk of KS may reflect the falling incidence of sexually transmitted diseases and thus the reduced likelihood of exposure to the causal agent.

There are no consistent racial differences in KS risk. Among homosexual and bisexual men with AIDS in the USA, white men have a higher risk of KS than black men (20% and 11%, respectively), whereas in the UK there is no difference in the risk by race (24% and 23%, respectively, for whites and blacks). The different risks for blacks and whites in the USA might well reflect behavioural factors.

It has been suggested that homosexual men with KS were more likely than others with AIDS to express HLA-DR5 (Goedert *et al*, 1987). Other studies did not confirm this finding but suggested instead an association with other HLA types. (These results are discussed in detail by Peterman *et al*, this issue.) Interpretation of these findings is complex given the marked geographical variations in KS risk.

Virological and Serological Studies

As it is now widely believed that a transmissible agent causes KS, laboratory studies hold the key to its identification. Serological studies of homosexual men with AIDS who have KS have, however, thus far yielded inconsistent and inconclusive findings. In most reports, a major problem has been that blood samples studied were obtained after the men developed AIDS. Since HIV associated immunosuppression increases susceptibility to infection, serological findings are difficult to interpret in people who already have AIDS. Moreover, men with KS are less severely immunosuppressed than are men with other manifestations of AIDS (Rabkin *et al*, 1990), and so they tend to have lower levels of antibodies to common infections than do men with other manifestations of AIDS. For example, Jacobsen *et al* (1990) found that just before the onset of AIDS, men with KS had lower levels of cytomegalovirus antibody than did men who presented with other opportunistic infections. They concluded that this was because the men with KS were less severely immunosuppressed than the other men.

Goedert *et al* (1987) reported serological findings for a small number of men whose blood had been stored before they were given a diagnosis of AIDS. They found that the men in whom KS developed had higher titres for hepatitis B surface antibody but not for other hepatitis antigens nor for antibodies to cytomegalovirus, Epstein-Barr virus or herpes simplex virus. Further studies of this sort are needed to identify which infections were common in people with KS before they developed AIDS.

KAPOSI'S SARCOMA ASSOCIATED WITH HETEROSEXUALLY ACQUIRED HIV INFECTION

Among AIDS patients, men and women who acquired HIV by heterosexual spread are, after homosexual and bisexual men, the group next most likely to have KS (Table 1). Just as with homosexual and bisexual men, the risk of KS varies considerably according to the country of origin of the individuals and the characteristics of their sexual partners.

Geographical Distribution

The risk of KS associated with heterosexually acquired HIV infection is especially high among men and women born or living in Africa or Caribbean countries. The proportion of AIDS patients reported to have KS ranges from 8% to 18% in people from Africa and from 6% to 9% in people from the Caribbean (Table 3). In contrast, 1% or fewer of those born in the USA or the UK who acquired HIV by heterosexual spread have KS. Before the AIDS epidemic, KS was comparatively common in certain areas of Africa. People from those areas may therefore be symptom free carriers of the causal agent, and HIV infection and its associated immunosuppression may well have resulted in the clinical expression of the disease. Little information is available about the incidence of KS in Caribbean countries before the advent of AIDS, except that it was more common in Puerto Rico than in the USA (Biggar et al, 1984). Thus the prev-

TABLE 3. Kaposi's sarcoma in AIDS patients who acquired HIV by heterosexual spread, by country of origin

Country of origin	AIDS subjects who have Kaposi's sarcoma reported
Africa	
Rwanda (Van der Perre et al, 1984)	18%
Zaire (Piot et al, 1984)	16%
Africa[a] (Beral et al, 1991)	14%
Zaire[b] (Clumeck et al, 1984)	13%
Africa[c] (Beral et al, 1990)	8%
Caribbean	
Caribbean countries other than Haiti[c] (Beral et al, 1990)	9%
Haiti[c] (Beral et al, 1990)	6%
USA/Europe	
USA (Beral et al, 1990)	1%
UK (Beral et al, 1991)	0%

[a]Resident in the UK
[b]Resident in Belgium
[c]Resident in the USA

alence of symptom free carriers may also have been higher in the Caribbean than in the US population before the spread of HIV, and this may account for the high risk of KS among people from the Caribbean.

Age, Sex, Race and Time Trends

There are no major differences in risk of KS by age or sex in the proportion of subjects with heterosexually transmitted HIV (Beral *et al*, 1990, 1991). For example, among Caribbean born people with AIDS who were living in the USA, 7% of the men and 5% of the women were reported to have KS, and among African heterosexuals with AIDS in the UK, 14% of both males and females were reported to have KS.

Most of those with KS and heterosexually acquired HIV infection are black or Hispanic, and this is likely to reflect the country of origin of the patients rather than racial susceptibility.

The proportion of heterosexuals with AIDS who also have KS has declined over time in the USA at a rate similar to that found in homosexual men (Beral *et al*, 1990). The reason is unclear.

Sexual Partners and Practices

Among women born in the USA who acquired HIV infection heterosexually, the major determinant of KS risk identified so far is whether their sexual partner was a bisexual male (Table 4). This suggests that among women the KS agent may well be acquired by sexual contact. Little else is known about the sexual partners or sexual practices of women with KS who acquired HIV by heterosexual spread.

KAPOSI'S SARCOMA ASSOCIATED WITH PARENTERALLY ACQUIRED HIV INFECTION

The risk of KS is low in individuals who acquired HIV infection parenterally—from infected needles, blood or blood products (see Table 1).

TABLE 4. Karposi's sarcoma risk in women born in the USA who acquired HIV by heterosexual contact, according to sexual partner's HIV transmission group[a]

Sexual partner's HIV transmission group	AIDS subjects who have Kaposi's sarcoma reported
Bisexual male	3.0%
Intravenous drug user	0.7%
Transfusion recipient or haemophiliac	0.0%

[a]From Beral *et al*, 1990

Geographical Distribution

Among individuals with AIDS who acquired HIV parenterally, KS was reported in 2.5% (509/20075) of the subjects in the USA, but not a single case has been reported in 293 subjects in the UK. The absence of KS in such populations in the UK is noteworthy and suggests that the causal agent may be less prevalent in the general UK population than in that of the USA.

Although information about individuals with parenterally acquired HIV infection is sparse, there is some evidence of geographical variations in KS risk within the USA that follow the variations in risk described for homosexual men. Among transfusion recipients and intravenous drug users with AIDS, for example, the risk of KS was highest in subjects living in California and New York, where KS was particularly common in homosexual men (Beral *et al*, 1990).

Few data are available from other countries except Spain and Italy, where the percentages of intravenous drug users with AIDS reported to have KS are similar to the percentage reported in the USA: 2.5% in Spain (Casabona *et al*, 1990) and 2.8% in Italy (Vaccher *et al*, 1989).

Other Factors

The risk of KS in individuals who acquired HIV parenterally is not related to age or sex but is higher in blacks than in whites (Beral *et al*, 1990).

KAPOSI'S SARCOMA IN CHILDREN WHO ACQUIRED HIV INFECTION PERINATALLY

Kaposi's sarcoma has been reported in children with AIDS from Africa, the Caribbean and Central America (Bouquety *et al*, 1989; Gutierrez-Ortega *et al*, 1989). Only 1% of children born in the USA who have perinatally acquired HIV infection are reported to have KS; all were the offspring of women who were born in the Caribbean (Beral *et al*, 1990). In the UK and Spain, no child with perinatally acquired HIV infection has been reported to have KS (Casabona *et al*, 1990; Beral *et al*, 1991).

The clinical manifestations of KS in young children are not the same as in adults, and diagnostic problems hamper comparisons (Scott *et al*, 1984). Nevertheless, existing evidence suggests that the risk of KS may be increased in children with AIDS whose parents come from African or Caribbean countries, where the incidence of KS was comparatively high before the AIDS epidemic. This suggests that the mothers might be symptom free carriers of the causal agent, which can be transmitted to an infant during the perinatal period.

INCUBATION PERIOD FOR KAPOSI'S SARCOMA IN HIV INFECTED PEOPLE AND SURVIVAL AFTER DIAGNOSIS OF AIDS

Kaposi's sarcoma is rarely a late complication of AIDS. In 80% of cases in which it occurs, KS is the presenting symptom (Lifson *et al*, 1990). Studies of transfusion recipients (Beral *et al*, 1990) and homosexual men (Lifson *et al*, 1990) have shown that the time between HIV infection and onset of AIDS is shorter for those with KS than for those with other manifestations of AIDS.

Survival was initially reported to be longer in homosexual men who presented with KS alone than in those with other opportunistic infections (Rothenberg *et al*, 1987). Recently this finding has not been confirmed (Payne *et al*, 1990). It is now clear that some homosexual and bisexual men who present with KS are not infected with HIV (Friedman-Kien *et al*, 1990). Before HIV was identified such men might have been classified as having AIDS and the benign course of their disease would have resulted in an apparently favourable survival for homosexual men with KS and no other illnesses.

CONCLUSIONS

There is growing evidence that all types of KS, whether associated with HIV infection or not, are caused by the same transmissible agent and that the clinical expression of the disease is determined by an individual's immune status.

Two unusual features of KS explain why a cluster of such a rare disease heralded the AIDS epidemic. Firstly there is now considerable evidence that the transmissible agent that causes KS is transmitted by sexual contact, as is HIV. Thus the circumstances that encouraged the spread of HIV and the explosive outbreak of AIDS also encouraged the spread of the KS agent. The second reason is that immunosuppression facilitates the clinical expression of KS in an otherwise symptom free carrier of the KS agent. Thus the immunosuppression caused by HIV in people who were carriers of the KS agent provided the opportunity for the disease to become manifest. The strange coincidence of the KS agent being spread in a similar way to HIV and of HIV associated immunosuppression resulting in the clinical expression of KS are probably the main reasons why KS is so extraordinarily common in people with AIDS.

Kaposi's sarcoma was a prominent feature of the early years of the AIDS epidemic in the USA and Europe but is becoming less common in people with AIDS as the epidemic spreads. One reason is that the AIDS epidemic initially affected homosexual men, who are at an especially high risk of developing KS. Moreover, KS tends to occur in the most sexually active homosexual men, who also tended to be among the first to develop AIDS. As the AIDS epidemic spreads to less sexually active homosexual men, their risk of developing KS is not as high. Furthermore, KS is now known to be an early manifestation of AIDS, occurring with relatively mild immunosuppression and usually being the presenting symptom of AIDS. Other manifestations of AIDS such as dementia are associated with severe immunosuppression and tend to occur late in the course of the disease. The subjects presenting with AIDS in the early years of the epidemic had been infected with HIV for a relatively short time, and it is not surprising that they presented with the conditions that occur early in the course of the illness.

Epidemiological studies have demonstrated that KS is rare among heterosexuals with AIDS from Europe or the USA but is relatively common in heterosexuals with AIDS from Africa or the Caribbean. The prevalence of the agent that causes KS is thus likely to be low in heterosexuals from Europe or the USA and high in heterosexuals from Africa or the Caribbean.

Present and future research is focusing on the mode of transmission of the KS agent and its identification. This is discussed in detail in Peterman *et al.* (this issue).

SUMMARY

The AIDS epidemic drew attention to KS, a previously rare and little studied condition. The epidemiological evidence summarized here strongly suggests that the disease is caused by a transmissible agent, in addition to HIV. Sexual contact is the most important mode of transmission of the agent, although transmission by blood and perinatally may also occur (Beral *et al*, 1990).

References

Abrams DI (1990) The relationship between KS and intestinal parasites among homosexual males in the United States. *Journal of Acquired Immune Deficiency Syndromes* **3** (**Supplement 1**) S44–S46

Archibald CP, Schechter MT, Craib KJP *et al* (1990) Risk factors for Kaposi's sarcoma in the Vancouver lymphadenopathy-AIDS study. *Journal of Acquired Immune Deficiency Syndromes* **3** (**Supplement 1**) S18–S23

Auerbach DM, Darrow WW, Jaffe HW and Curran JW (1984) Cluster of cases of the acquired immune deficiency syndrome. *American Journal of Medicine* **76** 487–492

Bayley AC, Downing RG, Cheingsong-Popov R, Tedder RS, Dalgleish AG and Weiss RA (1985) HTLV-III serology distinguishes atypical and endemic Kaposi's sarcoma in Africa. *Lancet* **i** 359–361

Bendsöe N, Dictor M, Blomberg J, Ågren S and Merk K (1990) Increased incidence of Kaposi's sarcoma in Sweden before the AIDS epidemic. *European Journal of Cancer* **26** 699–702

Beral V, Peterman TA, Berkelman RL and Jaffe HW (1990) Kaposi's sarcoma among persons with AIDS: a sexually transmitted infection? *Lancet* **335** 123–128

Beral V, Bull D, Jaffe H, Evans B, Gill N, Tillett H and Swerdlow AJ (1991) Risk of Kaposi's sarcoma in AIDS patients in the British Isles; is it increased if sexual partners come from the USA or Africa? *British Medical Journal* **324** 624–625

Biggar RJ, Horm J, Fraumeni JF Jr, Greene MH and Goedert JJ (1984) Incidence of Kaposi's sarcoma and mycosis fungoides in the United States including Puerto Rico, 1973–81. *Journal of the National Cancer Institute* **73** 89–94

Bouquety JC, Siopathis MR, Ravisse PR, Lagarde N, Georges-Courbot MC and Georges AJ (1989) Lympho-cutaneous Kaposi's sarcoma in an African pediatric AIDS case. *American Journal of Tropical Medicine and Hygiene* **40** 323–325

Casabona J, Salas T, Lacasa C, Melbye M and Segura A (1990) Kaposi's sarcoma in people with AIDS from an area in Southern Europe. *Journal of Acquired Immune Deficiency Syndromes* **3** 929–930

Casabona J, Melbye M, Biggar RJ and the AIDS registry contributors (1991) Kaposi's sarcoma and non-Hodgkin's lymphoma in European AIDS cases: no excess risk of Kaposi's sarcoma in Mediterranean countries. *International Journal of Cancer* **47** 49–53

Clumeck N, Sonnet J, Taclman H *et al* (1984) Acquired immunodeficiency syndrome in African patients. *New England Journal of Medicine* **310** 492–497

Darrow WW, Echenberg DF, Jaffe HW *et al* (1987) Risk factors for human immunodeficiency virus (HIV) infections in homosexual men. *American Journal of Public Health* **77** 479–483

Dörffel J (1932) Histogenesis of multiple idiopathic hemorrhagic sarcoma of Kaposi. *Archives of Dermatology and Syphilis* **26** 608–634

Friedman-Kien AE, Saltzman BR, Cao Y *et al* (1990) Kaposi's sarcoma in HIV-negative homosexual men. *Lancet* **i** 168–169

Giraldo G, Beth E and Haguenau F (1972) Herpes-type virus particles in tissue culture of Kaposi's sarcoma from different geographic regions. *Journal of the National Cancer Institute* **49** 1509–1526

Goedert JJ, Biggar RJ, Melbye M *et al* (1987) Effect of T4 count and cofactors on the incidence of AIDS in homosexual men infected with human immunodeficiency virus. *Journal of the American Medical Association* **257** 331–334

Gutierrez-Ortega P, Hierro-Orozco S, Sanchez-Cisneros R, Coyoacan A and Montano LF (1989) Kaposi's sarcoma in a 6-day old infant with human immunodeficiency virus. *Archives of Dermatology* **125** 432–433

Hansson CJ (1940) Kaposi's sarcoma: clinical and radiotherapeutic studies on twenty-three patients. *Acta Radiologica* **21** 457–470

Haverkos HW, Pinsky PF, Drotman P and Bregman DJ (1985) Disease manifestation among homosexual men with acquired immunodeficiency syndrome: a possible role of nitrites in Kaposi's sarcoma. *Sexually Transmitted Diseases* **12** 203–208

Hutt MSR (1984) Kaposi's sarcoma. *British Medical Bulletin* **40** 355–358

Jacobsen LP, Muñoz A, Fox R, Phair J, Dudley J, Obrams GI, Kingsley LA, Polk BF and the Multicentre AIDS cohort group (1990) Incidence of Kaposi's sarcoma in a cohort of homosexual men infected with the human immunodeficiency virus type 1. *Journal of Acquired Immune Deficiency Syndromes* **3** (**Supplement** 1) S24–S31

Jaffe H, Choi K, Thomas PA *et al* (1983) National case-control study of Kaposi's sarcoma and *pneumocystis carinii* pneumonia in homosexual men: Part 1, epidemiologic results. *Annals of Internal Medicine* **99** 145–151

Kaposi M (1872) Idiopathisches multiples pigmentsarkom der Haut. *Archiv Fur Dermatologie* **4** 265–273

Kinlen LJ (1982) Immunosuppressive therapy and cancer. *Cancer Surveys* **1** 565–583

Kitchen VS, French MAH and Dawkins RL (1990) Transmissible agent of Kaposi's sarcoma. *Lancet* **i** 797–798

Lifson AR, Darrow WW, Hessol NA *et al* (1990) Kaposi's sarcoma in a cohort of homosexual and bisexual men. *American Journal of Epidemiology* **131** 221–231

Mann DL, Murray C, O'Donnell M, Blattner WA and Goedert JJ (1990) HLA antigen frequencies in HIV-1-related Kaposi's sarcoma. *Journal of Acquired Immune Deficiency Syndromes* **3** (**Supplement** 1) S51–S55

Moss AR, Osmond D, Bacchetti P, Chermann J-C, Barne-Sinoussi F and Carlson J (1987) Risk factors for AIDS and HIV seropositivity in homosexual men. *American Journal of Epidemiology* **125** 1035–1047

Muret MPG, Soriano V, Pujol RM, Hewlett I, Clotet B and de Moragas JM (1990) AIDS and Kaposi sarcoma pre-1979. *Lancet* **i** 969–970

Oettle AG (1962) Geographical and racial differences in the frequency of Kaposi's sarcoma as evidence of environmental or genetic causes, In: Ackerman LV and Murray JF (eds). *Symposium on Kaposi's Sarcoma: Unio Internationalis Contra Cancrum* **18** 330–363, Karger, Basel

Payne SF, Lemp GF and Rutherford GW (1990) Survival following diagnosis of Kaposi's sarcoma for AIDS patients in San Francisco. *Journal of Acquired Immune Deficiency Syndromes* **3** (**Supplement** 1) S14–S17

Penn I (1988) Secondary neoplasms as a consequence of transplantation and cancer therapy.

Cancer Detection and Prevention **12** 39–57

Piot P, Quinn TC, Taelman H *et al* (1984) Acquired immunodeficiency syndrome in a heterosexual population in Zaire. *Lancet* **ii** 65–69

Polk BF, Fox R, Brookmeyer R *et al* (1987) Predictors of the acquired immunodeficiency syndrome developing in a cohort of seropositive homosexual men. *New England Journal of Medicine* **316** 61–66

Qunibi W, Akhtar M, Sheth K *et al* (1988) Kaposi's sarcoma: the most common tumor after renal transplantation in Saudi Arabia. *American Journal of Medicine* **84** 225–232

Rabkin CS, Goedert JJ, Biggar RJ, Yellin F and Blattner WA (1990) Kaposi's sarcoma in three HIV-1-infected cohorts. *Journal of Acquired Immune Deficiency Syndromes* **3** (**Supplement 1**) S38–S43

Ronchese F (1958) Kaposi's sarcoma: an overlooked essay of 1882. *AMA Archives of Dermatology* **77** 542–545

Ronchese F and Kern AB (1953) Kaposi's sarcoma (Angioreticulomatosis). *Postgraduate Medicine* **14** 101–111

Rothenberg R, Woelfel M, Stoneburner R, Milberg J, Parker R and Truman B (1987) Survival with the acquired immunodeficiency syndrome: experience with 5833 cases in New York City. *New England Journal of Medicine* **317** 1297–1302

Scott GB, Buck BE, Leterman JG, Bloom FL and Parks WP (1984) Acquired immunodeficiency syndrome in infants. *New England Journal of Medicine* **310** 76–81

Taylor JF, Smith PG, Bull D and Pike MC (1972) Kaposi's sarcoma in Uganda: geographic and ethnic distribution. *British Journal of Cancer* **26** 483–497

Vaccher E, Tirelli U, Lazzarin A *et al* (1989) Epidemic Kaposi's sarcoma in Italy, a country with intravenous drug abusers as the major group at risk for AIDS: a report of 60 cases. *AIDS* **3** 321

Vandenbroucke JP and Pardoel VPAM (1989) An autopsy of epidemiologic methods: the case of "poppers" in the early epidemic of the acquired immunodeficiency syndrome (AIDS). *American Journal of Epidemiology* **129** 455–457

Van de Perre P, Rouvroy D, Lepage P *et al* (1984) Acquired immunodeficiency syndrome in Rwanda. *Lancet* **ii** 62–65

The author is responsible for the accuracy of the references.

The Aetiology of Kaposi's Sarcoma

T A PETERMAN[1] • H W JAFFE[2] • A E FRIEDMAN-KIEN[3]
R A WEISS[4]

[1]Mailstop E02, Centers for Disease Control, Atlanta, Georgia 30333; [2]Mailstop G29, Centers for Disease Control, Atlanta, Georgia 30333; [3]Department of Dermatology and Microbiology, New York University Medical Center, New York, New York 10016; [4]Institute of Cancer Research, Royal Cancer Hospital, Chester Beatty Laboratories, London SW3 6JB

INTRODUCTION

Epidemiological evidence suggests that Kaposi's sarcoma (KS) is caused by an infectious agent whose expression is enhanced in an immunocompromised host (Beral, this issue). Identification of the putative infectious agent would lead to a better understanding of KS and perhaps to a means of preventing it. In this chapter, we will briefly review the pathophysiology of KS, its association with immunosuppression and what is known about the infectious agent. The focus will be on clues to the identity of the proposed infectious agent.

CLASSIFICATION OF KAPOSI'S SARCOMA: MANY PRESENTATIONS, ONE CAUSE?

Kaposi's sarcoma has been classified in many different ways, all of which have categories that are somewhat vague and overlap greatly. Clinically, KS has been divided into four types based on morphological presentation and biological behaviour: nodular, florid, infiltrative and lymphadenopathic. These four types were more relevant to African cases than to cases in Europe or North America (Safai and Good, 1981). Epidemiologically, KS has been classified into sporadic (classical), endemic (African), epidemic (AIDS related) and immunosuppression associated (usually transplant recipients). However, all clinical types of lesions can be seen in the endemic epidemiological class. Histologically, the four clinical types and four epidemiological types are often indistinguishable. In addition, cultured cells derived from classical and AIDS related KS appear to have identical immunohistochemical properties (Werner *et al*, 1989). Aetiologically, it seems most appropriate to consider KS as having one cause, with the clinical, histological and epidemiological characteristics dependent on the interaction between the putative KS transmissible agent and the immune system of the host.

PATHOPHYSIOLOGY[1]

Lesions

The clinical and histological picture of the KS skin lesions can vary within the same person. Many individuals have lesions in different stages of development at the same time. The early patch stage macular lesions contain abnormally shaped dilated vessels surrounded by a mononuclear cell infiltrate containing plasma cells; nuclear atypia and mitoses are rarely seen. In the plaque stage lesions, there is neoplastic proliferation in the superficial to deep dermis, with minimal proliferation of bundles of spindle shaped cells showing nuclear atypia and rare mitoses; extravasated red blood cells and deposits of haemosiderin are present. The more advanced nodular lesions contain a marked increase in fascicles of spindle cells which surround and compress the irregularly shaped vascular slits; sparse extravasated red blood cells are seen, and the mononuclear cell infiltrate is usually minimal (Safai, 1987; Silvers, 1989).

The histological appearance of the KS lesion is more consistent with "reactive hyperplasia" than with a malignant neoplasm (Costa and Rabson, 1983; Brooks, 1986). There is no well defined cluster of tumour cells. Lesions frequently appear in clusters in a widespread symmetrical distribution that is quite different from that seen in other sarcomas. Although cell cultures derived from AIDS related KS have shown a number of chromosomal rearrangements, they varied from culture to culture and even between cultures established from the same biopsy (Delli Bovi *et al*, 1986). Such chromosomal abnormalities are consistent with neoplasia, but few cells in mitosis were detected in fresh tumour cells, cell growth patterns did not appear transformed, the cells were not immortalized and they did not exhibit properties associated with transformation such as growing in soft agar medium or causing tumours in nude mice (Delli Bovi *et al*, 1986).

---

[1]See also Cockerell, this issue

Cells of Origin

Malignant neoplasms usually have an obviously abnormal cell type that can be considered the cell of origin. There are many cell types within a KS lesion, so it is difficult to determine a "cell of origin". Studies using various immunohistochemical stains of the cells within the KS lesions suggest they are similar to lymphatic endothelium, but this similarity is based more on the lack of staining for markers of vascular endothelium than on the presence of markers unique to lymphatic endothelium. The early abnormal vessels stained more like lymphatic endothelium than vascular endothelium using factor VIII related antigen, HLA-DR/Ia, macrophage/endothelial antigens, 5′ nucleotidase, ATPase, alkaline phosphatase and a lectin binder *Ulex europaeus I* (Beckstead *et al*, 1985). Staining of the spindle cell component of KS tissue with these stains was also consistent with the staining for lymphatic endothelium and two additional monoclonal antibodies, EN4 and PAL E (Jones *et al*, 1986). Both vascular endothelial cells and spindle cells in KS lesions are positive for the CD34 antigen, which is characteristic of bone marrow stem cells and vascular endothelium (Weiss, 1990). In all of these studies, it may be difficult to distinguish the abnormal spindle cells from the normal proliferating vessels within them. Furthermore, recent evidence has suggested that KS may not arise from endothelial cells at all but from dermal dendrocytes (Nickoloff and Griffiths, 1989).

Cultures from Kaposi's Sarcoma Lesions

Cells from KS lesions have been successfully grown in culture. Since there is no well defined KS cell, it is difficult to be certain that KS derived cell lines contain the true pathophysiological features of KS. Some of the cells that have been cultured have shown histological characteristics similar to the spindle shaped cells seen in KS lesions (Beckstead *et al*, 1985; Salahuddin *et al*, 1988). The growth of the KS cell cultures was enhanced by employing "conditioned media" harvested from cultures of T lymphocytes that were infected with human retroviruses, including human T lymphotropic virus (HTLV)-I, HTLV-II, HIV-1 and HIV-2 (Nakamura *et al*, 1988). The most potent stimulation of KS cells in vitro was found with media "conditioned" by HTLV-II; less stimulation was seen with HIV-1. The stimulation of KS cells by HTLV-II "conditioned media" was greater than the maximum stimulation from tested concentrations of interleukin-1, basic fibroblast growth factor (bFGF) and acidic fibroblast growth factor (aFGF), and the stimulation was not neutralized by antibodies to interleukin-1 or tumour necrosis factor alpha (TNFα). The AIDS related KS cells were established in long term culture using the "conditioned media" of HTLV-II infected lymphocytes. The KS cells themselves secreted substances that stimulate their growth or the growth of endothelial cells, including high levels of bFGF, interleukin-6 and interleukin-1-β and low levels of aFGF, interleukin-1-α and granulocyte-macrophage cell stimulating factor. There was no evidence of several other cytokines. Biological assays also showed very high levels of bFGF and interleukin-1 (Ensoli *et al*, 1989).

When cells cultured from AIDS related KS were transplanted onto chorioallantoic membrane of fertilized chicken eggs, they induced extensive vascularization. When the AIDS related KS cells were inoculated sub-cutaneously in nude mice, they induced transient vascular haemorrhagic lesions suggestive of the human KS lesions (Salahuddin *et al*, 1988).

Other investigators have maintained cultures of KS cells from classical lesions and found they had the same histological characteristics as cultures from AIDS related KS lesions (Delli Bovi *et al*, 1986). No evidence of tumorigenicity was found in soft agar culture or in nude mice. Both classical and AIDS related KS cells were strongly dependent on externally supplied growth factors.

Search for Oncogenes

Multiple oncogenes have been sought in the culture model, including c-*myc*, c-*fos*, c-N-*ras*, c-Ha-*ras*, c-*sis*, c-*fms* and c-*erb*B (Werner *et al*, 1989). There was no difference in oncogene expression between KS cells and fibroblasts from the KS patients. An oncogene has been identified following transfection of DNA from a KS lesion into NIH 3T3 cells (Lo and Liotta, 1985; Delli Bovi *et al*, 1987). The protein encoded by this oncogene is related to a fibroblast growth factor that has been shown to be mitogenic for fibroblasts and endothelial cells (Delli Bovi *et al*, 1988). The transformed 3T3 cells grew in serum free medium, consistent with an autocrine (self promoting) mechanism for growth. Although this oncogenic transformation would be an attractive explanation for the histological appearance of the KS lesions, this oncogene may have been generated during the gene transfer procedure (Delli Bovi and Basilico, 1987). The oncogene was not detectable in the original KS material, only one of several specimens produced a transforming colony and the same transforming oncogene has been identified by transfection of DNA from a human stomach cancer and from normal human stomach tissue (Sakamoto *et al*, 1986). This oncogene was not found in cultures of AIDS related KS cells (Ensoli *et al*, 1989).

IMMUNOSUPPRESSION THAT FACILITATES DISEASE EXPRESSION

It is probably correct to say that all types of KS are associated with some type of immunosuppression, although this immunosuppression may be difficult to identify in some persons. Kaposi's sarcoma has been associated with high rates of second malignancies, primarily lymphomas (Piette, 1987). A review of hospital records containing double primary malignancies showed a 20-fold increase in lymphoreticular malignancies after diagnosis of KS (Safai *et al*, 1980). A much smaller increase was detected using the Swedish Cancer Registry for 1958–1982; there were 13 KS associated lymphomas reported when only 5 were expected (Dictor and Attewell, 1988). For an individual patient there may be little evidence of immunosuppression. Some reports have mentioned decreased responses to skin testing in some African patients with KS (Taylor and Ziegler, 1974; Afrasiabi *et al*, 1986). One study reported tinea pedis in 40 of 40 patients with classical KS (Alteras *et al*, 1981). Classical KS is seen primarily in the elderly, possibly because of the same well recognized but poorly understood immune dysfunction that leads to reactivation of tuberculosis infection in older persons.

Some sort of malignancy develops in 6% of organ transplant recipients within a few years of beginning immunosuppressive therapy, and 3.5% of the malignancies are KS, suggesting a cumulative incidence of 0.2% (Penn, 1979). When immunosuppressive agents are discontinued, the KS often regresses and may disappear entirely. The most common immunosuppressive agents associated with KS are the corticosteroids used for renal transplant recipients. Kaposi's sarcoma has also been seen in recipients of other types of transplants as well as in persons receiving systemic corticosteroids for other conditions, including pemphigus, asthma, rheumatoid arthritis, biliary cirrhosis and nephrotic syndrome (Klepp *et al*, 1978). Since most of these are case reports, it is not possible to determine whether the incidence is higher or lower than in renal transplant recipients. Steroid therapy has also accelerated KS progression in some AIDS patients (Gill *et al*, 1989). Other immunosuppressive agents, including azathioprine and cyclosporin, have also been associated with KS, but rates are not known. Kaposi's sarcoma represents a higher proportion of the tumours reported for patients treated with cyclosporin (usually in combination with corticosteroids), but this may be a function of the duration of follow-up. Kaposi's sarcoma appears sooner after transplantation than do most other tumours, and patients treated with cyclosporin have a shorter follow-up time than patients treated with corticosteroids alone (Penn, 1987).

Major increases in the incidence of KS have accompanied the HIV epidemic. Our inability to identify the putative KS agent makes it impossible to determine whether AIDS represents a particularly supportive type of immunosuppression or whether there is an accompanying increase in KS "infection" in AIDS patients. In the beginning of the AIDS epidemic in the USA, 60% of the homosexual or bisexual men with AIDS had KS; thus at the level of immunosuppression seen with AIDS, KS lesions developed in 60–100% of those infected with the KS agent. Other HIV transmission categories such as intravenous drug users had a much lower risk of KS, but even in the lowest risk group KS was about ten times as common as in transplant recipients. There may be something about AIDS that is particularly efficient at facilitating the clinical expression of KS. Some laboratory evidence would support this. When the HIV *tat* gene was introduced into the germline of mice, multifocal skin lesions resembling KS lesions developed in male (but not female) offspring (Vogel *et al*, 1988). The mechanism by which the *tat* gene induces KS like vascular proliferations in transgenic mice is not known. Supernatants from HIV-1 infected H9 cells have promoted the growth of AIDS related KS cells in vitro, and antibody to the Tat protein prevented this stimulation (Ensoli *et al*, 1990). Recombinant Tat has the same properties.

For a while it was thought that the distribution of KS might be related to the distribution of HLA subtypes. An early study of patients with AIDS related KS found 12 (63%) of 19 patients had HLA DR5 compared with 53 (23%) of 231 community controls ($p<0.01$ after correcting for multiple comparisons) (Friedman-Kien *et al*, 1982). This association was interesting because the HLA DR5 allele is more common in Italians, blacks and Jews, in whom classical KS is also more likely to develop. This suggested that KS may be related to immune response genes linked to DR5. Another report seemed to confirm this link to DR5 in AIDS related and classical KS (Pollack *et al*, 1983). However, as additional patients with AIDS related KS were studied, this association between HLA DR5 and KS disappeared (Rubinstein *et al*, 1984). There have since been reports linking KS to HLA-A2 (Qunibi *et al*, 1988), -DR1, -DRw14, -DQw1 (Mann *et al*, 1988) and -A28 (Kuntz and Bruster, 1989).

The conditions associated with KS all suggest a disorder of cell mediated immunity. The more profound the disorder, the more rampant the KS. Kaposi's sarcoma is conspicuously absent from congenital disorders of cell mediated immunity, but this may reflect the rarity of congenital infection with the KS agent.

THE INFECTIOUS AGENT

Unprecedented reports of hundreds of persons with KS in sub-Saharan Africa led to the first international symposium on KS in 1961 in Kampala, Uganda (Hutt, 1984). At this symposium, it became apparent that KS was endemic in central Africa, with an uneven distribution centered in eastern Zaire where KS accounted for 10% of all malignancies (Hutt, 1984). It was during the early 1960s that Denis Burkitt first described the geographical distribution of an unusual lymphoma, and cultures of Burkitt's lymphoma led to the discovery of the Epstein-Barr virus (EBV), the first human tumour virus (Epstein, 1985). This undoubtedly influenced the search for a viral cause for KS. In 1972, cytomegalovirus (CMV), another herpesvirus, was detected in KS cell line cultures derived from African patients' tumours (Giraldo *et al*, 1972). Over the next 10–15 years, data accumulated to support the link between CMV and KS. Although CMV is no longer considered as the likely cause of KS, the evidence for and against that relationship is instructive in considering other possible aetiological agents.

Following the detection of CMV in the KS cell cultures, a number of serological studies were done. All of 16 Europeans with classical KS had detectable antibodies to CMV, compared with 31 (69%) of 45 controls, and the geometric mean CMV antibody titres were higher in the KS patients (Giraldo *et al*, 1975). Similar results were found for 30 Americans with KS (Giraldo *et al*, 1978). However, the CMV association was not seen in Africans with KS; all cases and controls had detectable antibody and their titres were similar (Giraldo *et al,* 1975, 1978).

Other observations also suggested that CMV might be the cause of KS. Acute CMV infection can cause a self limiting lymphoproliferative disorder. Cytomegalovirus frequently causes lifelong latent infections. It can persistently infect endothelial cell cultures and transform them to anchorage independent growth, an in vitro characteristic of neoplastic cells (Smiley *et al,* 1988). With the onset of the AIDS epidemic, CMV, which was already considered a sexually transmitted infectious agent in homosexual men, was suggested as the reason for the high prevalence of AIDS related KS in homosexual/bisexual men (Drew *et al,* 1982).

However, CMV is no longer thought to be the KS agent. In retrospect, several epidemiological aspects of KS in patients with AIDS spoke strongly against CMV, including the low prevalence of KS among intravenous drug users and haemophiliacs with AIDS, who are commonly infected with CMV. A variety of studies could not confirm that CMV infection was more common in persons with KS (Marmor *et al,* 1984). In more recent laboratory studies, CMV was often not found in KS lesions. Biopsy specimens from four of ten patients with AIDS related KS were found to be negative for CMV using four different techniques: immunohistochemical demonstration of CMV antigen, in situ hybridization, Southern blot and polymerase chain reaction gene amplification (van den Berg *et al,* 1989). Cytomegalovirus was detected in only 5 (20%) of 25 AIDS related KS lesions by in situ hybridization, and the CMV positive cells were few and sparsely distributed (Grody *et al,* 1988). In this same study, six lesions from patients with the classical form of KS had no evidence of CMV by DNA hybridization. Two of 13 AIDS related KS specimens hybridized to CMV DNA, but the CMV in the KS tissue seemed to be part of a generalized infection (Delli Bovi *et al,* 1986). Using specific CMV DNA probes, culture or electron microscopy, CMV was not detected in six AIDS related KS cell lines (Salahuddin *et al,* 1988). The transforming fragment of CMV, morphological transforming region II, which is present in CMV induced sarcomas seen in rodents, was not detected in the KS cell lines (Jahan *et al,* 1989). Taken together, these findings suggest that CMV may be a bystander in neoplastic tissue, existing either as a latent infection or reactivated by immunosuppressive therapy or by HIV infection.

Other known viruses have been looked for in patients with KS, in KS tissue and in KS cell lines. There has been no correlation with serological evidence of EBV, herpes simplex virus (HSV)-1, HSV-2 or hepatitis B virus (HBV) infection (Giraldo *et al,* 1978; Marmor *et al,* 1984). Likewise, there was no association of KS with detection of HBV, human herpesvirus (HHV)-6 or EBV in tissue biopsies (Jahan *et al,* 1989). The presence of other viruses has been unsuccessfully looked for in cell cultures derived from AIDS related KS cells, including HTLV-I, HTLV-II, HIV-1, HBV, HHV6, EBV, CMV, HSV-1, HSV-2, papova and polyoma viruses (Salahuddin *et al,* 1988). Although many of these viruses might be likely choices as a tumour associated virus, the distribution of these agents in the population is inconsistent with the distribution of KS. A novel, virus like infectious agent (which proved to be a mycoplasma) was obtained by direct transfection of DNA from KS tissue of an AIDS patient, but this same agent was found in many other sites and in AIDS patients who did not have KS (Lo *et al,* 1989).

The Clues

Evidence suggesting that an infectious agent is responsible for KS has accumulated rapidly with the onset of the transplant era and the AIDS epidemic. Kaposi's sarcoma has developed in many transplant recipients within a few weeks to months of starting therapy, suggesting that the progression from latent stage to disease can be rapid. On the other hand the predilection for KS in the elderly suggests that many could have been infected for decades before they manifest disease. This extremely long latent period may reflect a latent viral infection that becomes activated with the onset of immunosuppression. However, if such a quiescent infection is present, it must be unresponsive to the multiple chemotherapeutic agents taken by patients with AIDS before the onset of KS. An alternative mechanism would be that transformation occurs early after the KS agent infects the host, but the transformed cells are kept in check by the intact immune system.

There is a strong male predominance for some types of KS but not for others. The endemic form of KS in Africa and classical KS in the elderly clearly affect males more often than females (Beral, this issue). However, among transplant recipients and among AIDS patients (after stratifying by HIV transmission group) there is little if any male predominance (Penn, 1988; Beral *et al,* 1990). This variation in male predominance by type of KS may reflect differences in the distribution of immunosuppression, differences in the distribution of infection with the KS agent or both.

The routes of transmission for the KS agent are hard to trace because persons who are not immunosuppressed do not manifest the disease. Most transmission appears to be from symptom free persons. Despite our inability to identify the source of infection for an individual with KS, epidemiological studies of AIDS patients have demonstrated that airborne or casual transmission of the KS agent is unlikely and that sexual transmission is the most likely route (Beral *et al,* 1990). Homosexual men with AIDS were 20 times more likely to have KS than were haemophiliacs with AIDS. Women with AIDS who were sexual partners of bisexual men were more likely to have KS than women who were partners of intravenous drug users. Among homosexual men, there was an association with oral-anal contact, suggesting a possible faecal-oral agent (Jacobson *et al,* 1990). Transmission via blood is apparently less common, since KS was seen in only 2% of transfusion recipients even though 10–20% of them probably received blood from a donor who went on to develop KS. Even more striking is the paucity of cases among persons with haemophilia (1%) who had received clotting factor concentrates derived from thousands of donors and therefore had a high prevalence of past infection with HBV, CMV and other viruses. If the KS agent is present in blood, perhaps it is highly cell associated and/or inactivated during the preparation of factor concentrates. Perinatal transmission has been rarely reported, perhaps because so few HIV infected mothers are infected with the KS agent. A 6 week old boy developed AIDS related KS (Gutierrez-Ortega *et al,* 1989). His mother died of AIDS related toxoplasmosis a few weeks later, but no KS was found at necropsy, suggesting that even with AIDS, KS infections may be subclinical. Few other infants with AIDS related KS have been reported, and none of their mothers had developed AIDS by the time of those reports (Baum and Vinters, 1989).

There is some evidence that an epidemic of KS agent infection has occurred in the USA at about the same time as the epidemic of HIV infection (Friedman-Kien *et al,* 1990). In the USA, there have been reports over the period 1980 to 1990 of about 20 relatively young homosexual/bisexual men with KS who are not infected with HIV. Before the AIDS epidemic there were about 20 cases of KS per year in all men under age 50, including those who were immunosuppressed (Biggar *et al,* 1984). If there was an increase in KS in persons uninfected with HIV and the KS agent is transmitted by blood transfusion, there might be an increase in KS among transplant recipients in the USA. After excluding non-melanoma skin cancers and in situ cervical carcinomas, KS accounted for 4.9% of the tumours reported by 1979 and 5.9% of those added by 1988 (Penn, 1979, 1988). Some of this increase may be due to changes in which centres report tumours to the registry. A report from Saudi Arabia suggests that infection was quite common among transplant recipients between 1975 and 1986; 11 (4.2%) of 260 recipients being followed for post-transplant care (not just recipients with tumours) have developed KS (Qunibi *et al,* 1988). It is not clear whether this high frequency reflects a high prevalence of the KS agent in Saudis in general or a high frequency of transmission of the agent to the transplant recipients. Some of these persons had received their kidney transplants outside Saudi Arabia, and those who received transplants in Saudi Arabia may have received transfusions of blood imported from the USA (Harfi and Fakhry, 1986). A review of the Swedish cancer registry data from 1958 to 1982 suggested that the incidence of KS doubled in Sweden in the early 1960s (Dictor and Attewell, 1988). It is not clear how long the disease has been endemic in Africa. Reports were rare before 1942, possibly because cases were missed (Oettle, 1962).

The response of KS to various therapeutic interventions may also provide insight into the aetiology. As mentioned earlier, discontinuing immunosuppressive therapy such as corticosteroids often results in resolution of KS in the iatrogenically immunosuppressed host. Antibiotics and antimycobacterial therapy appear to be ineffective based on the absence of any reports of KS remission or resolution in AIDS patients with KS receiving antimicrobial therapy for other opportunistic infections. Antiviral agents, including those used for CMV retinitis such as foscarnet and ganciclovir, appear to be equally ineffective. In one study in which azidothymidine (AZT) treatment was given to 22 AIDS patients with stable KS, there was partial tumour regression in only two patients after 20 weeks (de Witt *et al*, 1989). Good responses of KS have been seen with interferon-α therapy given either systemically or intralesionally. Data are limited to phase II studies. One trial of high dose interferon-α (Roferon A) in 28 patients with AIDS related KS found a complete response in 5 patients and a partial response in 7 others, with response related to T4 count and stage of KS (de Witt *et al*, 1988). In this study, there were also increases in T4 counts and decreases in HIV antigen, so it was not clear whether the response of the patient's KS was due to improved immunological status or to a direct effect on the KS lesions. Another study found that the combination of interferon-α and AZT was associated with at least a partial response in 17 (46%) of 37 patients (Krown *et al*, 1990).

Although evidence is accumulating that interferon-α reduces KS growth, there are also data suggesting that other cytokines may facilitate KS growth. A phase II study of combined interleukin-2 and interferon-β was stopped after three of the first four patients had rapid progression of their KS, possibly because bolus injection of interleukin-2 increased production of interferon-γ (Krigel *et al*, 1989).

The Suspects

What type of agent should we look for as the cause of KS? In the 1960s, the EBV association with Burkitt's lymphoma made herpesviruses an obvious choice. In the 1980s, the boom in retrovirology made these viruses attractive candidates. Viruses other than retroviruses may be considered as alternatives, including enteric viruses such as rotaviruses or adenoviruses, especially since recent epidemiological evidence suggests that oral-faecal exposure may be a significant factor in the development of KS in homosexual men with AIDS.

Although the infectious cofactor for KS is most likely viral, another sort of transmissible agent is possible. For example, canine transmissible venereal tumour, a naturally occurring neoplastic disease of dogs, is thought to be spread by sexual transmission of a neoplastic cell (Cohen, 1985). Molecular biological studies have suggested that transmissible venereal tumour in various dogs has a common cell of origin (Katzir *et al*, 1987). If a similar pathogenic mechanism pertained to KS, it might be detected by examination of KS tissues for the presence of cells that are "foreign" to the host.

The authors (HWJ and RAW) tested this hypothesis by trying to detect Y chromosome specific DNA sequences in tumour specimens from women with KS. The detection method involved the use of a "nested" polymerase chain reaction procedure (Mullis and Faloona, 1987) to amplify a DNA sequence found in the pseudoautosomal boundary region of the human Y chromosome (Ellis *et al*, 1990). Although the method was sensitive enough to detect male DNA diluted 1/10 000 in female DNA, corresponding to approximately 100 pg of male DNA, no Y specific sequence could be detected in KS tissues of two

HIV infected African women. The hypothesis may therefore be incorrect, or alternatively, it could still be correct if the transmissible cell lacked this specific sequence, for example, the cell may be female in origin.

Further Investigation

The search for the proposed infectious agent of KS could retrace many of the steps that have already been taken using newer tests and different population groups. A general search for antibody to known infectious agents among patients with KS could identify associations with other agents that are transmitted in a similar fashion or perhaps detect cross-reactivity from the KS agent. Polymerase chain reaction technology could be used to search KS tissue for integrated genomic sequences of known viruses, and this may lead to the discovery of a new virus or a variant form of a known viral agent. Electron microscopy (EM) could be used to detect the presence of virus particles in KS tissue, but EM findings alone would be difficult to interpret. Other virus particles have been detected by EM but were not grown in culture (Rappersberger *et al*, 1990; Siegal *et al*, 1990). Kaposi's sarcoma lesions could be assayed for reverse transcriptase activity that should be present if retroviruses are replicating in the lesions. Attempts to culture KS tissue under different conditions may help facilitate the isolation of the KS agent. Kaposi's sarcoma lesions could be inoculated into immunosuppressed animals in an attempt to induce similar lesions in animals. There is an animal disease, avian haemangiomatosis, that shows some similarities to KS and is known to be caused by a retrovirus of the avian leukosis group (Dictor and Jarplid, 1988).

CONCLUSION

We do not know how long the discovery of the aetiology of KS will take, but the pace has accelerated in recent years. Understanding the aetiology of KS should ultimately facilitate the prevention and treatment of KS. Understanding the search for the aetiology of KS may help in the search for the causes of other diseases.

SUMMARY

The aetiology of KS remains unknown, but recent evidence suggests that the disease is caused by the presence of an infectious agent in an immunosuppressed host. Although there are a variety of clinical presentations, the putative infectious agent is likely to be the same in all cases. The pathophysiology of the lesions, the types of immunosuppression that facilitate disease expression, the response to therapy and the distribution of disease within immunosuppressed populations provide important clues to the nature of the unidentified infectious agent.

References

Afrasiabi R, Mitsuyasu RT, Nishanian P, Schwartz K and Fahey JL (1986) Characterization of a distinct subgroup of high risk persons with Kaposi's sarcoma and good prognosis who present with normal T4 cell number and T4:T8 ratio and negative HTLV-III/LAV serologic test results. *American Journal of Medicine* **81** 969–973

Alteras I, Cafri B and Feuerman EJ (1981) The high incidence of tinea and unguium in patients with Kaposi's sarcoma. *Pathologia* **74** 177–179

Baum LG and Vinters HV (1989) Lymphadenopathic Kaposi's sarcoma in a pediatric patient with acquired immune deficiency syndrome. *Pediatric Pathology* **9** 459–465

Beckstead JH, Wood GS and Fletcher V (1985) Evidence for the origin of Kaposi's sarcoma from lymphatic endothelium. *American Journal of Pathology* **119** 294–300

Beral V, Peterman TA, Berkelman RL and Jaffe HW (1990) Kaposi's sarcoma among persons with AIDS: a sexually transmitted infection? *Lancet* **335** 123–128

Biggar RJ, Horm J, Fraumeni JF Jr, Greene MH and Goedert JJ (1984) Incidence of Kaposi's sarcoma and mycosis fungoides in the United States including Puerto Rico, 1973–81. *Journal of the National Cancer Institute* **73** 89–94

Brooks JJ (1986) Kaposi's sarcoma: a reversible hyperplasia. *Lancet* **ii** 1309–1311

Cohen D (1985) The canine transmissible venereal tumor: a unique result of tumor progression. *Advances in Cancer Research* **43** 75–112

Costa J and Rabson AS (1983) Generalised Kaposi's sarcoma is not a neoplasm. *Lancet* **i** 58

Delli Bovi P and Basilico C (1987) Isolation of a rearranged human transforming gene following transfection of Kaposi's sarcoma DNA. *Proceedings of the National Academy of Science of the USA* **84** 5660–5664

Delli Bovi P, Donti E, Knowles DM II *et al* (1986) Presence of chromosomal abnormalities and lack of AIDS retrovirus DNA sequences in AIDS-associated Kaposi's sarcoma. *Cancer Research* **46** 6333–6338

Delli Bovi P, Curatola AM, Kern FG, Greco A, Ittmann M and Basilico C (1987) An oncogene isolated by transfection of Kaposi's sarcoma DNA encodes a growth factor that is a member of the FGF family. *Cell* **50** 729–737

Delli Bovi P, Curatola AM, Newman KM *et al* (1988) Processing, secretion, and biological properties of a novel growth factor of the fibroblast growth factor family with oncogenic potential. *Molecular and Cellular Biology* **8** 29

de Witt R, Schattenkerk JKME, Boucher CAB, Bakker PJM, Veenhof KHN and Danner SA (1988) Clinical and virological effects of high-dose recombinant interferon-α in disseminated AIDS-related Kaposi's sarcoma. *Lancet* **ii** 1214–1217

de Witt R, Reiss P, Bakker PJ, Lange JM, Danner SA and Veenhof KH (1989) Lack of activity of zidovudine in AIDS-associated Kaposi's sarcoma. *AIDS* **3** 847–850

Dictor M and Attewell R (1988) Epidemiology of Kaposi's sarcoma in Sweden prior to the acquired immunodeficiency syndrome. *International Journal of Cancer* **42** 346–351

Dictor M and Jarplid B (1988) The cause of Kaposi's sarcoma: an avian retroviral analog. *Journal of American Academy of Dermatology* **18** 398–402

Drew WL, Conant MA, Miner RC *et al* (1982) Cytomegalovirus and Kaposi's sarcoma in young homosexual men. *Lancet* **ii** 125–127

Ellis N, Taylor A, Bengtsson BO, Kidd J, Rogers J and Goodfellow P (1990) Population structure of the human pseudoautosomal boundary. *Nature* **344** 663–665

Ensoli B, Nakamura S, Salahuddin SZ, Biberfeld P, Larsson L, Beaver B, Wong-Staal F and Gallo RC (1989) AIDS-Kaposi's sarcoma-derived cells express cytokines with autocrine and paracrine growth effects. *Science* **243** 223–226

Ensoli B, Barillari G, Salahuddin SZ, Gallo RC and Wong-Staal F (1990) Tat protein of HIV-1 stimulates growth of cells derived from Kaposi's sarcoma lesions of AIDS patients. *Nature* **345** 84–86

Epstein MA (1985) Historical background: Burkitt's lymphoma and Epstein-Barr virus, In: Lenoir GM, O'Connor GT and Olwney CLM (eds). *A Human Cancer Model: Burkitt's*

Lymphoma, pp 17–27, Oxford University Press, New York

Friedman-Kien AE, Laubenstein LJ, Rubinstein P *et al* (1982) Disseminated Kaposi's sarcoma in homosexual men. *Annals of Internal Medicine* 96 693–697

Friedman-Kien A, Saltzman BR, Cao Y *et al* (1990) Kaposi's sarcoma in HIV-negative homosexual men. *Lancet* 335 168–169

Gill PS, Loureiro C, Bernstein-Singer M, Rarick MU, Sattler F and Levine AM (1989) Clinical effect of glucocorticoids on Kaposi's sarcoma related to the acquired immunodeficiency syndrome (AIDS). *Annals of Internal Medicine* 110 937–940

Giraldo G, Beth E and Haguenau F (1972) Herpes-type virus particles in tissue culture of Kaposi's sarcoma from different geographic regions. *Journal of the National Cancer Institute* 49 1509–1513

Giraldo G, Beth E, Kourilsky FM *et al* (1975) Antibody patterns to herpesviruses in Kaposi's sarcoma: serological association of European Kaposi's sarcoma with cytomegalovirus. *International Journal of Cancer* 15 839–848

Giraldo G, Beth E, Henle W, Henle G *et al* (1978) Antibody patterns to herpesviruses in Kaposi's sarcoma. II. Serological association of American Kaposi's sarcoma with cytomegalovirus. *International Journal of Cancer* 22 126–131

Grody WW, Lewin KJ and Naeim F (1988) Detection of cytomegalovirus DNA in classic and epidemic Kaposi's sarcoma by in situ hybridization. *Human Pathology* 19 524–528

Gutierrez-Ortega P, Hierro-Orozco S, Sanchez-Cisneros R and Montano LF (1989) Kaposi's sarcoma in a 6-day-old infant with human immunodeficiency virus. *Archives of Dermatology* 125 432–433

Harfi HA and Fakhry BM (1986) Acquired immunodeficiency syndrome in Saudi Arabia: the American-Saudi connection. *Journal of the American Medical Association* 255 383–384

Hutt MSR (1984) Kaposi's sarcoma. *British Medical Bulletin* 40 355–358

Jacobson LP, Munoz A, Fox R, Phair JP, Dudley J, Obrams GI, Kingsley F and The Multicenter AIDS Cohort Study Group (1990) Incidence of Kaposi's sarcoma in a cohort of homosexual men infected with human immunodeficiency virus type 1 *Journal of Acquired Immune Deficiency Syndromes* 3 Suppl 1 S24–S31

Jahan N, Razzaque A, Greenspan J *et al* (1989) Analysis of human KS biopsies and cloned cell lines for cytomegalovirus, HIV-1, and other selected DNA virus sequences. *AIDS Research and Human Retroviruses* 5 225–231

Jones RR, Spaull J, Spry C and Jones EW (1986) Histogenesis of Kaposi's sarcoma in patients with and without acquired immune deficiency syndrome (AIDS). *Journal of Clinical Pathology* 39 742–749

Katzir N, Arman E, Cohen D, Givol D and Rechavi G (1987) Common transmissible venereal tumors (TVT) in dogs. *Oncogene* 1 445–448

Klepp O, Dahl O and Stenwig JT (1978) Association of Kaposi's sarcoma and prior immunosuppressive therapy: a 5-year material of Kaposi's sarcoma in Norway. *Cancer* 42 2626–2630

Krigel RL, Padavic-Shaller KA, Rudolph AR, Poiesz BJ and Comis RL (1989) Exacerbation of epidemic Kaposi's sarcoma with a combination of interleukin-2 and β-interferon: results of a phase 2 study. *Journal of Biological Response Modifiers* 8 359–365

Krown SE, Gold JWM, Neidzwiecki D *et al* (1990) Interferon-α with zidovudine: safety, tolerance, and clinical and virologic effects in patients with Kaposi sarcoma associated with the acquired immunodeficiency syndrome (AIDS). *Annals of Internal Medicine* 112 812–821

Kuntz BM and Bruster HT (1989) Time-dependent variation of HLA-antigen-frequencies in HIV-1-infection (1983-1988). *Tissue Antigens* 34 164–169

Lo SC and Liotta LA (1985) Vascular tumors produced by NIH/3T3 cells transfected with human AIDS Kaposi's sarcoma DNA. *American Journal of Pathology* 118 7–13

Lo SC, Shih JW, Yang NY, Ou CY and Wang RY (1989) A infectious agent in patients with AIDS. *American Journal of Tropical Medicine and Hygiene* 40 213–226

Mann DL, Murray C, Yarchoan R, Blattner WA and Goedert JJ (1988) HLA frequencies in HIV-1 seropositive disease-free individuals and patients with AIDS. *Journal of Acquired Immune Deficiency Syndromes* **1** 13–17

Marmor M, Friedman-Kien AE, Zolla-Pazner S *et al* (1984) Kaposi's sarcoma in homosexual men: a seroepidemiologic case-control study. *Annals of Internal Medicine* **100** 809–815

Mullis KS and Faloona FA (1987) Specific synthesis of DNA in vitro via polymerase-catalyzed chain reaction. *Methods in Enzymology* **155** 335–350

Nakamura S, Salahuddin SZ, Biberfeld P *et al* (1988) Kaposi's sarcoma cells: long-term culture with growth factor from retrovirus-infected CD4+ T cells. *Science* **242** 426–443

Nickoloff BJ and Griffiths CEM (1989) The spindle-shaped cells in cutaneous Kaposi's sarcoma: histologic simulators include factor XIIIa dermal dendrocytes. *American Journal of Pathology* **135** 793–800

Oettle AG (1962) Geographical and racial differences in the frequency of Kaposi's sarcoma as evidence of environmental or genetic causes. *Acta Union Internationale Contra Cancrum* **18** 330–363

Penn I (1979) Kaposi's sarcoma in organ transplant recipients. *Transplantation* **27** 8–11

Penn I (1987) Cancers following cyclosporine therapy. *Transplantation* **43** 32–35

Penn I (1988) Secondary neoplasms as a consequence of transplantation and cancer therapy. *Cancer Detection and Prevention* **12** 39–57

Piette WW (1987) The incidence of second malignancies in subsets of Kaposi's sarcoma. *Journal of American Academy of Dermatology* **16** 855–861

Pollack MS, Safai B, Myskowski PL, Gold JWM, Pandey J and Dupont B (1983) Frequencies of HLA and Gm immunogenetic markers in Kaposi's sarcoma. *Tissue Antigens* **21** 1–8

Qunibi W, Akhtar M, Sheth K, Ginn HE, Al-Furayh O and DeVol EB (1988) Kaposi's sarcoma: the most common tumor after renal transplantation in Saudi Arabia. *American Journal of Medicine* **84** 225–232

Rappersberger K, Tschachler E, Zonzits E *et al* (1990) Endemic Kaposi's sarcoma in human immunodeficiency virus type 1-seronegative persons: demonstration of retrovirus-like particles in cutaneous lesions. *Journal of Investigative Dermatology* **95** 371–381

Rubinstein P, Rothman WM and Friedman-Kien A (1984) Immumologic and immunogenetic findings in patients with epidemic Kaposi's sarcoma. *Antibiotics and Chemotherapy* **32** 87–98

Safai B (1987) Pathology and epidemiology of epidemic Kaposi's sarcoma. *Seminars in Oncology* **14 (Supplement 3)** 7–12

Safai B and Good RA (1981) Kaposi's sarcoma: a review and recent developments. *CA-a Cancer Journal for Clinicians* **31** 2–12

Safai B, Mike V, Giraldo G, Beth E and Good RA (1980) Association of sarcoma with second primary malignancies: possible etiopathogenic implications. *Cancer* **45** 1472–1479

Sakamoto H, Mori M, Taira M *et al* (1986) Transforming gene from human stomach cancers and a noncancerous portion of stomach mucosa. *Proceedings of the National Academy of Sciences of the USA* **83** 3997–4001

Salahuddin SZ, Nakamura S, Biberfeld P *et al* (1988) Angiogenic properties of Kaposi's sarcoma-derived cells after long-term culture in vitro. *Science* **242** 430–433

Siegal B, Levinton-Kriss S, Schiffer A *et al* (1990) Kaposi's sarcoma in immunosuppression: possibly the result of a dual viral infection. *Cancer* **65** 492–498

Silvers DN (1989) The microscopic diagnosis of classical and epidemic AIDS-associated Kaposi's sarcoma, In: Friedman-Kien A (ed). *Color Atlas of AIDS*, pp 71–82, WB Saunders Company, Philadelphia

Smiley ML, Mar E-C and Huang E-S (1988) Cytomegalovirus infection and viral-induced transformation of human endothelial cells. *Journal of Medical Virology* **25** 213–226

Taylor JF and Ziegler JL (1974) Delayed cutaneous hypersensitivity reactions in patients with Kaposi's sarcoma. *British Journal of Cancer* **30** 312–318

van den Berg F, Schipper M, Jiwa M, Rook R, van de Rijke F and Tigges B (1989) Implausibility of an aetiological association between cytomegalovirus and Kaposi's sarcoma shown by four techniques. *Journal of Clinical Pathology* **42** 128–131

Vogel J, Hinrichs SH, Reynolds RK, Luciw PA and Jay G (1988) The HIV *tat* gene induces dermal lesions resembling Kaposi's sarcoma in transgenic mice. *Nature* **335** 606–611

Weiss RA (1990) The conundrum of Kaposi's sarcoma. *European Journal of Cancer* **26** 657–659

Werner S, Hofschneider PH and Roth WK (1989) Cells derived from sporadic and AIDS-related Kaposi's sarcoma reveal identical cytochemical and molecular properties in vitro. *International Journal of Cancer* **43** 1137–1144

The authors are responsible for the accuracy of the references.

Clinical Aspects of Epidemic Kaposi's Sarcoma

A BUCHBINDER • A E FRIEDMAN-KIEN

New York University Medical Center, New York, New York 10016

INTRODUCTION: PERSPECTIVE OF EPIDEMIC KAPOSI'S SARCOMA

Classical Kaposi's Sarcoma

Kaposi's sarcoma (KS), an unusual neoplastic disorder first described by Moritz Kaposi in 1872 (Kaposi, 1872), is a tumour that was found mostly in men over 50 years of age of Jewish and Italian descent. The male to female ratio was about ten to one (Oettle, 1962; Rothman, 1962; DiGiovanni and Safai, 1981). The clinical manifestations of this rare "classical" form of the disease have been well defined: a benign, indolent disease often limited to the lower extremities. Patients usually present with one or more violaceous flat to nodular lesions (occurring in clusters if more than one). With time, involvement of distant skin sites, lymph nodes, gastrointestinal tract and other organs may occur. As the disease progresses the lesions may coalesce and develop into larger nodules. Such lesions may become ulcerated and infected. Impairment of lymphatic or venous drainage is common, with resulting chronic oedema of the legs. Pain, discomfort, ulceration or invasion of underlying tissues often requires palliative treatment such as local radiation therapy, laser surgery, excision, intralesional injection of chemotherapeutic agents or electrocautery and curettage (Friedman-Kien *et al*, 1989). When widespread mucocutaneous involvement or symptomatic spread to visceral organ involvement occurs, systemic chemotherapy may be needed. Approximately one-third of patients with classical KS develop a second malignancy, most often non-Hodgkin lymphoma (Safai *et al*, 1980).

African Endemic Kaposi's Sarcoma

In the 1940s, more aggressive forms of KS were described in Africa, primarily in young adults, with a male to female ratio of ten to one (Oettle, 1962; Rothman, 1962). In Uganda, KS was found to account for 9% of all cancers (Oettle, 1962). The incidence of KS in the white and Asian populations living in regions of endemic KS was found to be low, similar to the incidence of classical KS in North America and Europe (Hood *et al*, 1980).

Four distinct variants of the endemic African form of KS have been described: (a) a benign nodular type that resembles the classical localized indolent disease; (b) an aggressive form, characterized by large, fungating and infiltrating skin lesions that are reported to respond to radiation therapy but that commonly invade underlying subcutaneous soft tissues and bone causing irreversible damage; (c) a rapidly and widely disseminated florid type of disease with local invasion, early visceral involvement and poor survival; and (d) a rare and virulent lymphadenopathic form with widespread lymph node involvement, seen predominantly in prepubescent black children, with a male to female ratio of three to one (Davies and Loethe, 1962; Taylor *et al*, 1971; Templeton and Bhana, 1975; Friedman-Kien *et al*, 1989). Retrospective serological studies for HIV antibodies performed on stored patient sera have demonstrated that these four forms of endemic African KS were not related to HIV infection (H. Jaffe, personal communication).

Recently, a cluster of 12 elderly patients with KS has been described in the Peloponese and southern Greece in whom the clinical course resembles that seen in African endemic KS. Eight men and four women aged 48 to 80 displayed multiple KS lesions in all stages of development. The lesions were most pronounced on the distal parts of the lower and upper extremities but also occurred more proximally and on the head, neck and face. Upper gastrointestinal lesions were present in nine patients, and one-third had indolent palpable lymph nodes in the inguinal and cervical regions. A retrovirus like particle was found on electron microscopy of the tumours, although all the patients were found to be seronegative for HIV by enzyme linked immunosorbent assay (ELISA) and Western blot. The patients were not incapacitated by the KS lesions (Kaloterakis, 1984; Rappersberger *et al*, 1990).

Kaposi's Sarcoma in Iatrogenically Immunosuppressed Patients

In the 1970s, cases of KS were found to occur in about 3% of iatrogenically immunosuppressed patients who had undergone renal transplantation. The lesions were in many cases limited to the skin, but with occasional widespread skin dissemination and involvement of visceral organs (Myers *et al,* 1974; Stribling *et al,* 1978; Hanid *et al,* 1989). Immunosuppressive therapy with corticosteroids was especially associated with this form of KS, and in many cases the KS lesions disappeared when the immunosuppressive therapy was discontinued, reduced or changed (Klein *et al,* 1974; Leung *et al,* 1981). Although the disease has been found to be limited to the skin and mucous membranes in two-thirds of the patients, prognosis is poor in the one-third in whom visceral involvement develops. The KS lesions appear a median of 16 months after the onset of immunosuppressive therapy, and a male to female ratio of between two and three to one has been reported (Klein *et al,* 1974).

Epidemic Kaposi's Sarcoma

In the early 1980s, an epidemic of a fulminant and disseminated form of KS was observed among sexually active young homosexual or bisexual men in New York and California (Friedman-Kien, 1981; Friedman-Kien *et al,* 1981; Gottlieb *et al,* 1981a; Hymes *et al,* 1981). The clinical manifestations of KS in this group together with the simultaneous occurrence of *Pneumocystis carinii* pneumonia in otherwise healthy homosexual men (Friedman-Kien, 1981; Gottlieb *et al.,* 1981b) served to define a previously unrecognized severe type of AIDS now known to be caused by infection with a retrovirus, HIV, first isolated in 1983. The clinical manifestations of KS associated with AIDS will now be described, together with a brief discussion of another recently described potentially epidemic form of KS not associated with HIV infection.

CLINICAL MANIFESTATIONS OF EPIDEMIC KAPOSI'S SARCOMA

Kaposi's sarcoma is an AIDS related disease most prevalent in patients whose risk factor for HIV infection is male homosexual behaviour, accounting for 95% of all AIDS associated KS. It is rarely found in AIDS patients with other HIV risk factors, ie intravenous drug abusers and recipients of HIV tainted blood or blood products (such as haemophiliacs). The falling incidence of KS from 1981 to 1990 in homosexual men is possibly related to remarkable modifications of high risk sexual behaviour, which have also led to a significant reduction in the incidence of HIV infection in this population. In 1981, about 48% of homosexual men with AIDS presented with or developed KS during the course of their illness. The incidence of AIDS related KS in 1990 in this population was less than 15%, but 95% of all AIDS related KS is still found among homosexual men. The remaining cases of AIDS related KS have been in intravenous drug users, a few transfusion recipients who incidentally received blood from homosexual men (in about 20% of whom KS developed during the course of their disease) and a few women partners of bisexual men. The clinical characteristics of KS variants are summarized in Table 1.

Associated with this decrease in HIV associated KS has been an increase in

TABLE 1. Clinical characteristics of Kaposi's sarcoma variants[a]

Type	Predominant mucocutaneous lesions	Mucocutaneous distribution	Lymph node involvement	Visceral involvement	Behaviour
Classical	Some patches, mostly plaques and nodules, usually rounded	Usually confined to lower extremities; disseminated lesions late in course of disease	Rare	Occasional	Indolent—gradual increase in number of lesions, often associated with lymphoedema; visceral lesions occur late, often discovered at necropsy; survival 10 to 15 years
Endemic African benign nodular	Papules and nodules	Multiple localized tumours, most commonly seen on lower extremities	Rare	Rare	Indolent, resembles classical type disease; survival 8 to 10 years
aggressive	Large exophytic nodules and fungating tumours	Most often located on the extremities	Rare	Occasional	Progressive development of multiple lesions with invasion and destruction of underlying tissue and bone; survival 5 to 8 years

florid	Nodules	Widely disseminated	Occasional	Occasional	Rapidly progressive; locally aggressive and invasive, early visceral involvement; survival 3 to 5 years
lymphadenopathic	Rarely manifests lesions	Minimal	Always	Frequent	Rapidly progressive; survival 2 to 3 years
Iatrogenic immunosuppression	Patches, plaques and nodules	Usually localized to the extremities; rarely disseminated	Rare	Occasional	Indolent; occasional tumour regression after immunosuppressive therapy is discontinued
Epidemic HIV associated	Patches, plaques, nodules; often fusiform and irregular	Multifocal, widely disseminated, often symmetrical; oral lesions common	Frequent	Frequent	Rapidly progressive; survival 2 months to 5 years
Non-HIV associated	Patches and plaques	Few small multifocal	Rare	Rare	Indolent course; survival up to 18 years

[a]Adapted from Friedman-Kien, 1989

the number of sexually active young homosexual men in whom a benign form of KS has developed but who have repeatedly been shown to have no laboratory or clinical evidence of immunosuppression. These men have been found not to be infected with HIV by the most reliable laboratory methods currently available, including serological testing with ELISA and Western blot, p24 antigenaemia, polymerase chain reaction (PCR) of their peripheral blood lymphocytes (PBL) with HIV specific primers and culture of PBL for HIV or reverse transcriptase activity. Although the diagnosis of AIDS should be entertained in any individual at high risk for HIV infection with KS, it is important that laboratory evidence of HIV infection, including serological status, be carefully confirmed before a diagnosis of AIDS is made in patients with KS and risk factors for HIV infection, since the presence of "epidemic" KS should no longer be regarded as synonymous with or necessarily diagnostic of AIDS.

In Africa, where HIV appears to be heterosexually transmitted and where men and women are equally affected by AIDS, the prevalence of epidemic KS associated with AIDS is reported to be equal in men and women (Beral, this issue). As described above, other forms of KS are more prevalent in males.

Mucocutaneous Manifestations

Kaposi's sarcoma may be present in almost any organ in patients with AIDS, but the most common locations include the skin, mucous membranes, lymph nodes and gastrointestinal tract. Except for the presence of KS lesions, the majority of those patients presenting with mucocutaneous KS are otherwise symptom free. Although KS lesions may be the first manifestation of HIV infection, tumours may appear at any time in the course of the disease—sometimes after the development of one or more life threatening opportunistic infections. The prognosis and survival of patients with KS are correlated with the absolute number of helper T lymphocytes in the blood, with systemic "B" symptoms such as fever, malaise, significant weight loss, diarrhoea and thrush; and with the development of one or more opportunistic infections. KS is rarely the cause of death in AIDS patients (Chachoua et al, 1989).

The KS lesions are often multifocal, widely disseminated and symmetrically distributed along the lines of skin cleavage (Langer's lines) (Fig. 1). Oral lesions are frequently present (Gaglioti et al, 1989). Early KS lesions appear as asymptomatic pink to deep purple or brown patches (Fig. 2), often elongated, oval, fusiform or irregular in shape, that may be overlooked for months by the patient or the physician. The flat macular lesions can develop into elevated plaques or nodules (Figs. 3 and 4), which sometimes coalesce to form a large nodular mass (Friedman-Kien and Saltzman, 1990). Lesions that appear on areas of the skin such as the occipital region and the earlobes and lesions of the buccal mucosa such as the palate or oropharynx may go undetected (Friedman-Kien, 1990a). Some patients have involvement of lymph nodes or visceral organs in the absence of mucocutaneous KS.

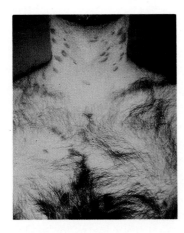

Fig. 1. Epidemic KS, plaque stage. A 26 year old homosexual male with widespread symmetrical cutaneous patches and nodules. Many of the lesions appear to follow the creases of the skin (Langer's lines).

Fig. 2. Epidemic KS, patch stage. A dark, violet patch appearing on the hard palate of a homosexual male. Such lesions are almost always asymptomatic and may not be noticed by the patient.

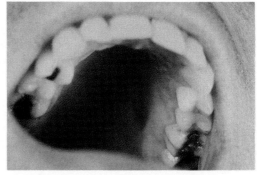

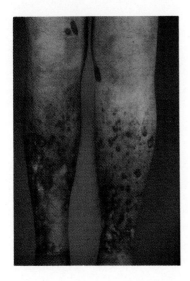

Fig. 3. Epidemic KS, plaque stage. Confluent raised dark brown plaques, predominantly located on the lower extremities, evolved in this middle aged homosexual male of Mediterranean origin. Chronic lymphoedema developed, with symptoms requiring radiation therapy. Radiation atrophy, hyper and hypopigmentation are apparent.

Fig. 4. Epidemic KS, patch to plaque stage. Mauve lesions are present on the glans of this 34 year old male. Lesions may be visible only on retraction of the foreskin.

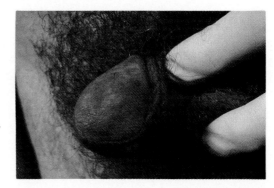

Throughout the course of the disease new lesions will appear that arise de novo and are not metastatic from other existing lesions. Only in its end stage does KS act as a truly malignant tumour, with aggressive behaviour and the development of metastases. This aspect of KS was noted by Kaposi himself in his original description of the disease and is well illustrated in epidemic KS.

Differential diagnosis of KS varies with the stage of the skin lesion. The flat, patch stage (Fig. 2) may simulate bruises, purpura, venous lakes, haemangiomas, pigmented naevi or malignant melanoma. Plaques can resemble pityriasis rosea, secondary syphilis, lichen planus, insect bites, papular urticaria, sarcoidosis, urticaria pigmentosa, intradermal naevi, malignant melanoma, basal cell carcinoma, squamous cell carcinoma or cutaneous metastases of internal malignancies. Nodular stage KS lesions (Fig. 3) can resemble dermatofibromas, pyogenic granulomas, neurofibromas, haemangiomas, angiosarcomas, fibrosarcomas, basal cell carcinomas, malignant melanoma and cutaneous metastases from systemic malignancies (Friedman-Kien and Ostreicher, 1984; Friedman-Kien and Saltzman, 1990).

Almost all AIDS patients with KS ultimately develop disseminated disease with lymph node and visceral organ involvement. The site of involvement and the tumour load do not correlate with prognosis (Safai et al, 1985). The development of pleuropulmonary KS is an ominous sign and occurs especially in AIDS patients whose deaths are directly attributed to KS (Ognibene et al, 1985; Meduri et al, 1986; Gill et al, 1989).

Pulmonary Manifestations

Estimates of the incidence of pulmonary KS vary with the methods used to diagnose KS. A large, multicentre clinical study found clinical evidence of pulmonary KS in 36 of 1067 (3.4%) patients with known or suspected AIDS and pulmonary symptoms (Murray et al, 1984), whereas post-mortem evidence of KS was found in 20–50% of AIDS patients (Reichert, 1983; Guarda et al, 1984; Nash and Fligiel 1984; Welch et al, 1984). Pulmonary KS occurs most frequently in the setting of disseminated disease but is sometimes discovered only at necropsy. In one large study of AIDS patients with pulmonary symptoms, all patients with pulmonary KS also had pulmonary infections (Murray et al, 1984). Kaposi's sarcoma was infrequently diagnosed by bronchoscopy but was found more frequently on open lung biopsies and at necropsy (Murray et al, 1984). Tumour involvement of the lung varies from interstitial infiltrates in alveolar walls and bronchovascular sheaths to nodular masses obliterating the underlying pulmonary tissue (Nash and Fligiel, 1984). In an evaluation of patients with mucocutaneous or lymphadenopathic KS, 30 of 66 patients developed pulmonary disease (Ognibene et al, 1985). Pulmonary KS was diagnosed in 12, with 6 patients diagnosed at necropsy. Open lung biopsies were required for the diagnosis. Neither the duration, the extent or the stability of mucocutaneous or lymphadenopathic KS was a useful indicator of pulmonary

KS. In 6 of the 30 patients, KS was the only cause of the pulmonary symptoms.

The symptoms of pulmonary KS are non-specific, patients often presenting with fevers, dyspnoea and associated X ray abnormalities. The chest radiogram shows soft shadows, reticulonodular shadows or pleural effusions or may even be normal. Thus KS should be ruled out as a cause of pulmonary symptoms or radiographic abnormality in patients with AIDS. Although the diagnosis may be established by fibreoptic bronchoscopy and endobronchial biopsy, where the lesions appear most commonly as diffuse erythematous or violaceous plaques, the patchy nature of the tumour, the absence of specific tumour markers and crush artifacts make open lung biopsies sometimes necessary for diagnosis (Pass *et al*, 1984; Ognibene *et al*, 1985; Hamm *et al*, 1987; Hanson *et al*, 1987).

Kaposi's sarcoma has also been described in the larynx in one patient with progressive vocal weakness who had disseminated cutaneous as well as oral KS (Levy and Tansek, 1990).

Gastrointestinal Manifestations

Kaposi's sarcoma frequently affects the gastrointestinal tract in patients with AIDS. Approximately 40% of patients with cutaneous KS have gastrointestinal involvement, and no correlation was found between gastrointestinal involvement and lymphadenopathic or oral KS in patients with cutaneous KS (Rose *et al*, 1982; Friedman *et al*, 1985) nor was survival affected by the presence of gastrointestinal KS (Friedman *et al*, 1985). Usually, cutaneous lesions are present before the diagnosis of gastrointestinal KS, but KS may present initially in the gut and is found there in 20–50% of patients at post-mortem (Reichert *et al*, 1983; Guarda *et al*, 1984; Welch *et al*, 1984). The symptoms that accompany KS are non-specific, and many patients are free of symptoms. Complaints of rectal pain, bleeding, diarrhoea or signs of occult bleeding, rectal masses and, rarely, massive bleeding may occur. In patients without known gastrointestinal involvement with KS, atypical presentations such as rectal bleeding due to KS involving the ileum (Neff *et al*, 1987), ulcerative colitis complicated by toxic megacolon (Biggs *et al*, 1987), rectal ulcer (Endean *et al*, 1987) and even simulating haemorrhoids (Khan *et al*, 1989) have been described. Kaposi's sarcoma lesions may be present in the oesophagus, stomach, small bowel, colon or rectum. The tumours predominantly involve the submucosa, with later involvement of the mucosa and sometimes also the deeper layers of the bowel wall (Biggs *et al*, 1987).

At endoscopy, typical KS lesions are described as vascular looking umbilicated nodules, as pigmented papules or as a telangiectasia that can vary in size from several millimetres to more than 1 cm. More advanced nodular lesions may be ulcerated, and some KS lesions have been described as having an "elephant skin" appearance (Friedman-Kien *et al*, 1982; Bernal *et al*, 1985; Cosnes *et al*, 1986). Since submucosal involvement is most common, diagnostic biopsies should include this layer (Biggs *et al*, 1987). Although a KS lesion may have a vascular appearance, the tumour rarely bleeds excessively unless it is attached to a larger blood vessel which becomes eroded. Radiological studies are not helpful in detecting macular KS lesions, although they may reveal KS plaques and tumour nodules (Rose *et al*, 1982).

Involvement of Visceral Organs

At necropsy, KS has often been found to involve a variety of internal organs and anatomical locations not discussed above, including the mediastinum (23%), liver (10–40%), retroperitoneum (23%), pericardium and epicardium (10–15%), seminal vesicles and epididymis (10–15%), urinary bladder (8%) and bone marrow (8%) (Reichert *et al*, 1983; Guarda *et al*, 1984; Welch *et al*, 1984; Friedman *et al*, 1985). Splenic, pancreatic, adrenal and intraluminal aortic KS have also been reported (Welch *et al*, 1984; Friedman *et al*, 1985). The lesions found at necropsy are frequently very small and do not appear to have contributed to the patient's death. When KS has been related to the cause of death, extensive involvement of multiple organs is usually present. The central nervous system and testes are rarely if ever involved with KS.

Non-HIV Related Epidemic Kaposi's Sarcoma

Increasing numbers of KS cases are now being reported in otherwise healthy homosexual men in the USA and Europe who have no laboratory or clinical evidence of HIV infection by ELISA, Western blot, p24 antigenaemia, viral culture or PCR (Afrasiabi *et al*, 1986; Marquart, 1986; Archer *et al*, 1989; Dictor and Bendsöe, 1990; Friedman-Kien *et al*, 1990; Garcia-Muret *et al*, 1990; Kitchen *et al*, 1990). These patients do not have any evidence of immune deficiency. No symptoms or signs referable to other organs have been noted, and investigation of visceral involvement has not been warranted. In these individuals, the disease appears as one or more small, biopsy proved KS skin lesions that can be found anywhere on the body. The course of the disease does not appear to be aggressive, and the removal of the tumour at the time of diagnosis has, after long term follow-up, been curative (Friedman-Kien *et al*, 1990). Patients treated with radiation therapy or local surgical therapy have had no recurrences, and one patient (Kitchen *et al*, 1990), a bisexual man, remained untreated without progression for 18 years. Kaposi's sarcoma should be part of the differential diagnosis of any suspicious macular, plaque, vascular or nodular pigmented lesions in sexually active individuals.

SUMMARY

Whereas previously KS represented a very rare and obscure neoplasm, it has become over the past decade a significant disease. Its appearance in various well defined risk populations and in immunosuppressed individuals and the mounting epidemiological evidence that KS may well represent a sexually transmitted disease in certain groups make KS an important tumour to study as a model for carcinogenesis. Among the various forms of KS described, it is the epidemic form of KS, most frequently associated with HIV infection, that is now the most prevalent form seen around the world. Clinically, the mucocutaneous and lymph node involvement are its most frequently recognized manifestations. Skin lesions in epidemic KS, unlike those in classical KS, appear anywhere on the skin or oral mucosa and at any age in patients with AIDS. Visceral lesions are often present, sometimes in the absence of cutaneous KS. Epidemic KS is rarely the cause of death in AIDS patients, even in those with visceral involvement, unlike the HIV-1 unrelated African endemic form of KS, which is an aggressive and malignant tumour. HIV testing is necessary to establish the diagnosis of AIDS in patients with epidemic KS, even in those patients with risk factors for HIV infection, since epidemic KS may represent an epidemic disease caused by a yet unidentified transmissible agent distinct from HIV. Concurrent transmission of HIV and the putative "KS agent" may have occurred in the homosexual patients with AIDS in whom KS has been so prevalent, and the recently identified form of epidemic KS in individuals not infected with HIV may well become yet a new form of this curious disease.

Acknowledgements

Support for this work was obtained from the Howard Gilman Foundation, the Saram Chait Memorial Foundation, NYU-CFAR, and the VA RCAHI. We give credit to William Slue (Division of Photography, Department of Dermatology, NYU Medical Center) for taking the photographs.

References

Afrasiabi R, Mitsuyasu RT and Nishanian P (1986) Characterization of a distinct subgroup of high risk persons with Kaposi's sarcoma and good prognosis who present with normal T4 cell number and T4:T8 ratio and negative HTLVIII/LAV serologic test results. *American Journal of Medicine* **81** 969–973

Archer CB, Spittle MF and Smith NP (1989) Kaposi's sarcoma in a homosexual––10 years on. *Clinical and Experimental Dermatology* **14** 233–236

Bernal A, del Junco GW and Gibson SR (1985) Endoscopic and pathologic features of gastrointestinal Kaposi's sarcoma: a report of four cases in patients with the acquired immune deficiency syndrome. *Gastrointestinal Endoscopy* **31** 74–77

Biggs BA, Crowe SM, Lucas CR, Ralston M, Thompson IL and Hardy KJ (1987) AIDS related Kaposi's sarcoma presenting as ulcerative colitis and complicated by toxic megacolon. *Gut* **28** 1302–1306

Chachoua A, Krigel RL, Lafleur F *et al* (1989) Prognostic factors and staging classifications of patients with epidemic Kaposi's sarcoma. *Journal of Clinical Oncology* **7** 774–780

Cosnes J, Darmoni SJ, Evard D and Le Quintrec Y (1986) Interet des explorations endoscopiques digestives au cours du syndrome d'immunodepression acquise. *Annales de*

Gastroenterologie et d'Hépatologie **22** 123–128

Davies JNP and Loethe F (1962) Kaposi's sarcoma in African children. *Acta Union Internationale Contra Cancrum* **18** 394–399

Dictor M and Bendsöe N (1990) Transmissible agent of Kaposi's sarcoma. *Lancet* **335** 797

DiGiovanni JJ and Safai B (1981) Retrospective study of 90 cases with particular emphasis on the familial occurrence, ethnic background and prevalence of other diseases. *American Journal of Medicine* **71** 779–783

Endean ED, Ross CW and Strodel WE (1987) Kaposi's sarcoma appearing as a rectal ulcer. *Surgery* **101** 767–769

Friedman SL, Wright TL and Altman DF (1985) Gastrointestinal Kaposi's sarcoma in patients with acquired immunodeficiency syndrome. *Gastroenterology* **89** 102–108

Friedman-Kien AE, Laubenstein L, Marmor M *et al* (1981) Kaposi's sarcoma and pneumocystis pneumonia among homosexual men—New York and California. *Morbidity and Mortality Reports* **30** 305–308

Friedman-Kien, AE (1981) Disseminated Kaposi-like sarcoma syndrome in young homosexual men. *Journal of the American Academy of Dermatology* **5** 468–470

Friedman-Kien AE and Ostreicher R (1984) Overview of classical and epidemic Kaposi's sarcoma, In: Friedman-Kien AE and Laubenstein LJ (eds). *AIDS: The Epidemic of Kaposi's Sarcoma and Opportunistic Infections*, pp 235–239, Masson Publishing, New York

Friedman-Kien AE and Saltzman BR (1990) Clinical manifestations of classical, endemic African, and epidemic AIDS-associated Kaposi's sarcoma. *Journal of the American Academy of Dermatology* **22** 1237–1250

Friedman-Kien AE, Laubenstein LJ, Rubinstein P *et al* (1982) Disseminated Kaposi's sarcoma in homosexual men. *Annals of Internal Medicine* **96** 693–700

Friedman-Kien AE, Ostreicher R and Saltzman BR (1989) Clinical manifestations of classical, endemic African, and epidemic AIDS-associated Kaposi's sarcoma, In: Friedman-Kien AE (ed). *Color Atlas of AIDS*, pp 11–48, WB Saunders Company, Philadelphia

Friedman-Kien AE, Saltzman BR, Cao Y *et al* (1990) Kaposi's sarcoma in HIV negative homosexual men. *Lancet* **335** 168–169

Gaglioti D, Ficara G, Nardi P and Mazzotta F (1989) Sarcoma di Kaposi orale: spettro clinico e istopatologico. *Minerva Stomatologica* **38** 1143–1150

Garcia-Muret MP, Soriano M, Pujol RM, Hewlett I, Clotet B and DeMoragas JM (1990) AIDS and Kaposi's sarcoma pre-1979. *Lancet* **335** 969–970

Gill PS, Akil B, Colletti P *et al* (1989) Pulmonary Kaposi's sarcoma: clinical findings and results of therapy. *American Journal of Medicine* **87** 57–61

Gottlieb GJ, Ragaz A, Vogel JV *et al* (1981a) A preliminary communication on extensively disseminated Kaposi's sarcoma in young homosexual men. *American Journal of Dermatopathology* **3** 111–114

Gottlieb MS, Schroff R, Schanker HM *et al* (1981b) *Pneumocystis carinii* pneumonia and mucosal candidiasis in previously healthy homosexual men: evidence of a new acquired immunodeficiency. *New England Journal of Medicine* **305** 1425–1431

Guarda LA, Luna MA, Smith L, Mansell PWA, Gyorkey F and Roca AN (1984) Acquired immune deficiency syndrome: postmortem findings. *American Journal of Clinical Pathology* **81** 549–557

Hamm PG, Judson MA and Aranda CP (1987) Diagnosis of pulmonary Kaposi's sarcoma with fiberoptic bronchoscopy and endobronchial biopsy: a report of five cases. *Cancer* **59** 807–810

Hanid MA, Suleiman M, Haleem A, Al Karaei M and Al Khader A (1989) Gastrointestinal Kaposi's sarcoma in renal transplant patients. *Quarterly Journal of Medicine* **73** 1143–1149

Hanson PJV, Harcourt-Webster JN, Gazzard BG and Collins JV (1987) Fiberoptic bronchoscopy in diagnosis of bronchopulmonary Kaposi's sarcoma. *Thorax* **42** 269–271

Hood AF, Farmer ER and Weiss RA (1980) Kaposi's sarcoma. *Bulletin Johns Hopkins Medical Journal* **151** 222–230

Hymes K, Cheung T, Greene JB *et al* (1981) Kaposi's sarcoma in homosexual men. *Lancet* **ii** 598–600

Kaloterakis A (1984) Kaposi's sarcoma in Greece. (Mediterranean Kaposi's sarcoma). Thesis, University of Athens, 1984

Kaposi M (1872) Idiopatiches multiples pigment sarcom der Haut. *Archiv fur Dermatologie Syphilis* **4** 265–272

Khan AA, Ravalli S, Vincent RA and Chabon AB (1989) Primary Kaposi's sarcoma simulating hemorrhoids in a patient with acquired immune deficiency syndrome. *American Journal of Gastroenterology* **84** 1592–1593

Kitchen VS, French AH and Dawkins RL (1990) Transmissible agent of Kaposi's sarcoma. *Lancet* **335** 798

Klein MB, Pereira FA and Kantor I (1974) Kaposi's sarcoma complicating systemic lupus erythematosus treated with immunosuppression. *Archives of Dermatology* **110** 602

Leung F, Fam AG and Osoba D (1981) Kaposi's sarcoma complicating corticosteroid therapy for temporal arteritis. *American Journal of Medicine* **71** 320–322

Levy FE and Tansek KM (1990) AIDS-associated Kaposi's sarcoma of the larynx. *Ear, Nose and Throat Journal* **69** 177–184

Marquart KH, Oehlschlaegel G and Engst R (1986) Disseminated Kaposi's sarcoma that is not associated with acquired immunodeficiency syndrome in a bisexual man. *Archives of Pathology and Laboratory Medicine* **110** 346–347

Meduri GU, Stover DE, Lee M, Myskowski PL, Caravelli JF and Zaman MB (1986) Pulmonary Kaposi's sarcoma in the acquired immune deficiency syndrome. *American Journal of Medicine* **81** 11–18

Murray JF, Felton CP, Garay SM *et al* (1984) Pulmonary complications of the acquired immunodeficiency syndrome. *New England Journal of Medicine* **310** 1682–1688

Myers BD, Kessler E, Levi J, Pick A and Rosenfeld J (1974) Kaposi's sarcoma in kidney transplant recipients. *Archives of Internal Medicine* **133** 307–310

Nash G and Fligiel S (1984) Pathologic features of the lung in the acquired immune deficiency syndrome (AIDS): an autopsy study of seventeen homosexual males. *American Journal of Clinical Pathology* **81** 6–12

Neff R, Kremer S, Voutsinas L, Waxman M and Mitty W (1987) Primary Kaposi's sarcoma of the ileum presenting as massive rectal bleeding. *American Journal of Gastroenterology* **82** 276–277

Oettle AG (1962) Geographical and racial differences in the frequency of Kaposi's sarcoma as evidence of environmental or genetic causes. *Acta Union Internationale Contra Cancrum* **18** 330–363

Ognibene FP, Steis RG, Macher AM *et al* (1985) Kaposi's sarcoma causing pulmonary infiltrates and respiratory failure in the acquired immunodeficiency syndrome. *Annals of Internal Medicine* **102** 471–475

Pass HI, Potter DA, Macher AM *et al* (1984) Thoracic manifestations of the acquired immune deficiency syndrome. *Journal of Thoracic and Cardiovascular Surgery* **88** 654–658

Rappersberger K, Tschachler E, Zonzits E *et al* (1990) Endemic Kaposi's sarcoma in human immunodeficiency virus type 1-seronegative persons: demonstration of retrovirus-like particles in cutaneous lesions. *Journal of Investigative Dermatology* **95** 371–381

Reichert CM, O'Leary TJ, Levens DL, Simrell CR and Macher AM (1983) Autopsy pathology in the acquired immune deficiency syndrome. *American Journal of Pathology* **112** 357–382

Rose HS, Balthazar EJ, Megibow AJ, Horowitz L and Laubenstein LJ (1982) Alimentary tract involvement in Kaposi sarcoma: radiographic and endoscopic findings in homosexual men. *American Journal of Radiology* **13** 661–666

Rothman S (1962) Some clinical aspects of Kaposi's sarcoma in the European and North American population. *Acta Union Internationale Contra Cancrum* **18** 364–371

Safai B, Mike V, Giraldo G, Beth E and Good RA (1980) Association of Kaposi's sarcoma with secondary primary malignancies: possible etiopathogenic implications. *Cancer* **45** 1472–

1479

Safai B, Johnson KG, Myskowski PL *et al* (1985) The natural history of Kaposi's sarcoma in the acquired immunodeficiency syndrome. *Annals of Internal Medicine* **103** 744–750

Stribling J, Wertzner S and Smith GC (1978) Kaposi's sarcoma in renal allograft recipients. *Cancer* **42** 442–446

Taylor JF, Templeton AC and Vogel CL (1971) Kaposi's sarcoma in Uganda: a clinicopathological study. *International Journal of Cancer* **8** 125–135

Templeton AC and Bhana D (1975) Prognosis in Kaposi's sarcoma. *Journal of the National Cancer Institute* **5** 1301–1304

Welch K, Finkbeiner W, Alpers CE *et al* (1984) Autopsy findings in the acquired immune deficiency syndrome. *Journal of the American Medical Association* **252** 1152–1154

The authors are responsible for the accuracy of the references.

Occurrence, Clinical Behaviour and Management of Kaposi's Sarcoma in Zambia

A C BAYLEY

Department of Surgery, University of Zambia, PO Box 32379, Lusaka, Zambia

Introduction
    Recognition of a new disease pattern
    Increasing incidence: implications for management
Clinical pattern
    Demographic features and HIV seropositivity
    Onset, progression and regression
    Weight loss and lymphadenopathy
    Oral and gut lesions
    Skin lesions, oedema and infiltration
    Pleural effusions and pulmonary infiltration
    Opportunistic infections
    Is HIV related Kaposi's sarcoma a true sarcoma?
Management
    Diagnosis and investigation
    Prognostic factors and staging
    To treat or not to treat?
    Actinomycin D and vincristine
    Phase II trial of epirubicin with vincristine
    Adjuncts to chemotherapy
    Decentralization of management to district hospitals
    Effects on the family and care in the home
Conclusions
Summary

INTRODUCTION

Recognition of a New Disease Pattern

Thirty years ago endemic Kaposi's sarcoma (KS), a chronic disease of skin and subcutaneous tissues, was recognized in middle aged men living in the equatorial belt of Africa. Endemic KS attracted attention for several reasons. Firstly, the geographical distribution suggested an environmental cause. Next, disease behaviour was curious: spontaneous regression of lesions was recorded quite often by reliable observers, and the illness pursued an indolent course for many years before terminating fatally. Finally, lesions were invariably multiple, with no evidence of spread from a single primary site, and they had a unique distribution (for a malignant tumour) on the most distal parts of one or more limbs. Early observers considered whether these clinical features and the reactive histology reflected an inflammatory process due to fungal or bacterial infection, rather than a neoplastic one. After failing to find a causative microorganism in tissue sections, they decided that endemic KS was a malignant tumour of mesodermal origin but of uncertain cell type (Ackerman *et al*, 1962).

The clinical features of endemic KS were: mean age at diagnosis about 40 years; male sex dominant in a ratio of at least 10:1; and multiple, nodular and sometimes ulcerated lesions with centrifugal distribution, preceded and accompanied by hot oedema. General health was well maintained during an indolent course lasting several years before more aggressive growth and central spread. Defects in cellular immunity were demonstrated only in patients who had reached this terminal phase, but at any stage in the process treatment with one or two of several cytotoxic drugs (vincristine, actinomycin D, dacarbazine [DTIC], bleomycin, razoxane, carmustine [BCNU] and adriamycin) could effect rapid disappearance of tumour masses, sometimes leaving fibrotic contractures of joints that were previously encased in hot infiltrated tissues (Olweny, 1981; Vogel, 1981). Radiotherapy was known to be effective but was rarely available in countries with a high incidence of endemic KS. When surgery was used for biopsy (in the event of drug failure or to reduce the size of troublesome masses) rapid and complete epithelialization of an incision through tumour tissue was often seen. The cell of origin remained a matter for debate; Hutt suggested that lesions arose from pluripotent vasoformative cells that differentiated towards several cell types (endothelium, fibroblasts and myofibroblasts) within tumours (Hutt, 1981).

Endemic KS was less common in Zambia than in Uganda, and between 1977 and 1982 I saw 8 to 12 new patients each year in Lusaka. In 1983, the number of patients with a histological diagnosis of KS doubled, but half of these patients had unfamiliar signs, including symmetrical lymphadenopathy, oral and gastrointestinal disease, gross weight loss and even absence of skin lesions from limbs. Although all 10 patients with classical signs responded to chemotherapy and were alive at the end of the year, 8 of 13 in the group with atypical signs failed to maintain initial responses to treatment and died before the end of 1983 (Bayley 1984). In 1984, the number of new patients with an atypical disease pattern increased, and most had antibodies in their blood to a newly described human T lymphotropic retrovirus, now known as HIV-1. When tested, patients had abnormal ratios of helper to suppressor lymphocytes, analogous to those observed in men with the new disease AIDS in the West. In 1984, only 2% of 158 Zambian controls (mean age 35 years) had antibodies in their blood, and none of 123 recently delivered mothers in Lusaka were seropositive, suggesting that the virus was newly introduced into Zambia at that time (Bayley *et al*, 1985).

Increasing Incidence: Implications for Management

Figure 1 shows the numbers of new patients with HIV related KS seen in Lusaka annually since 1982. In August 1990, 5 to 8 new patients presented each week, suggesting that over 300 new patients should be recorded by the end of 1990. Extension of this exponential curve suggests that there may be over a thousand new patients with KS each year in Lusaka alone by 1995.

In the past, the management of malignant tumours with chemotherapy has been regarded as a specialist field restricted to doctors with appropriate training and best avoided by those working in district hospitals. If cytotoxic drug treatment is genuinely useful to patients with KS, then this traditional opinion deserves re-examination.

In my opinion, the behaviour of HIV related KS in Africa is at least as strange as that of endemic KS, particularly when it coexists with HIV infection for several years. I believe that this strangeness invites us to reopen the question that exercized clinicians and pathologists in Uganda 30 years ago: is this disease a malignant tumour, or is it not?

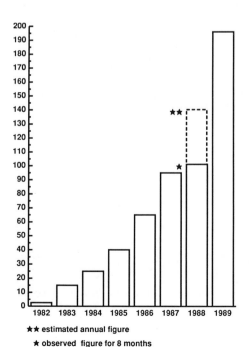

★★ estimated annual figure

★ observed figure for 8 months

Fig. 1. Numbers of new patients with HIV related KS in Lusaka, 1982–1989

CLINICAL PATTERN

Demographic Features and HIV Seropositivity

HIV related KS occurs more commonly in women than endemic disease, but it is still predominantly a disorder of men, with a sex ratio of M:F=5:1. However, this overall ratio hides an uneven distribution of women in the different clinical stages (which will be described below). Fewer than 10% of new patients in Lusaka have disease confined (apparently) to lymph nodes, and in this small group the sex ratio is nearly equal (M:F=1.7:1). The sex ratio at the next stage is 2.9:1, contrasting with a ratio of 9:1 among patients with the most advanced manifestations. There is no obvious explanation for these discrepancies.

In two studies (of 196 consecutive patients [Bayley, 1988] and a drug trial [Bayley, 1990]) men were older than women at diagnosis. Men present at a mean age of 35 years (range 13 to 56) and women at a mean age of 28 years (range 4 to 58).

In the early stages of the epidemic, patients with HIV related KS appeared to be better off economically and educationally than men with endemic KS, who were usually labourers or subsistence farmers. With time, this socio-economic difference has diminished, and patients are now drawn from all sections of society.

In a review of 196 patients with KS seen in Lusaka between 1982 and 1987 (Bayley, 1988), 143 of 150 examined had antibodies to HIV (95.3%), in contrast with 8 of 39 (20%) in sera from men with endemic KS, a figure which corresponds to the seroprevalence in adults admitted to an intensive care unit in Lusaka (Watters et al, 1988).

In Zambia, HIV is transmitted mainly by heterosexual activity or vertically from mother to fetus and to a small extent by blood or unsterilized skin piercing instruments. This determines the family circumstances of new patients with KS. Many have an HIV infected spouse, who may be ill also, and in many cases the youngest child has died or is sick at home.

Onset, Progression and Regression

Patients with endemic KS have a mean duration of symptoms of 17 months before presentation, but those with HIV related disease average only 8 months (Bayley, 1988). Some patients describe an acute onset of symptoms in terms such as those used by patients with appendicitis or pneumonia; as I have seen for myself, skin lesions may appear or spread over 12 to 48 hours.

As in endemic KS, spontaneous regression of lesions is seen in patients with HIV related KS, although this is very rare. For example, I saw some skin plaques disappear, while others developed, in a patient with early disease who declined treatment, but the most striking instance of regression was in a man with advanced KS that had ceased to respond to available chemotherapy.

Weight Loss and Lymphadenopathy

Weight loss and lymphadenopathy are the most common presenting symptoms of new patients with KS in Lusaka, occurring in 76% and 71%, respectively. These two signs are not linked, and patients who present with lymphadenopathy alone form a subgroup of particular interest.

We do not know how often KS tissue is confined to nodes, because this is a chance finding. In one study by a colleague (Bem C, personal communication) 9 of 100 consecutive HIV positive patients having node biopsies had a histological diagnosis of KS, as did 13% of 218 patients undergoing node biopsies without HIV testing during the same period.

Most patients with a histological diagnosis of KS who do not have skin or oral lesions are symptom free, except for discomfort from their node masses, which may be very large, particularly in the neck and groins. They have not lost weight and are muscular, with healthy hair and skin. When nodes are very large, I give one or two doses of vincristine, which often reduces their size, and then withhold treatment to wait for the development of new signs. A group reported in 1988 (Bayley, 1988) had a median observation period of 25 months for patients successfully followed up, but 2 of 11 are known to have died (at 1 and 10 months from diagnosis), and one was ill when last seen at 9 months, so the prognosis is not uniformly good. All patients tested for antibodies to HIV were seropositive.

Weight loss is an unambiguous finding strongly linked to prognosis in the 1988 survey (Bayley, 1988). Weight loss was recorded as gross when it was known or estimated to exceed 10 kg. A third of all patients had gross weight loss, and 42% of these died at a median of 1 month (range <1 to 9 months) from diagnosis, in contrast with a mortality of 27% in patients without weight loss at a median of 6 months (range 3 to 19 months) from diagnosis.

Oral and Gut Lesions

Oral lesions are more common than skin lesions and were seen in 58% of patients in Lusaka (see also Buchbinder and Friedman-Kien, this issue), sometimes in association with oral hairy leukoplakia or candidiasis. Throughout 1984, Din (personal communication) performed flexible endoscopy of the upper gastrointestinal tract on all patients with a clinical diagnosis of KS of either type. With one exception, only patients who had visible lesions in the mouth had multiple red or purple nodules protruding into the oesophagus, stomach or duodenum, although the submucous location of these lesions made proof of their histology by biopsy a rare event. Similarly, proctoscopy was positive for Kaposi like nodules whenever it was done, although I have known only one patient in 8 years who had rectal symptoms (mild bleeding and prolapse). The few necropsies that have been done have shown that patients with oral KS also have lesions throughout the gut, yet we have seen only two patients with intussusception needing surgery (Khorshid et al, 1987).

Oral lesions occur most commonly on the hard palate, adjacent to the gingival ridge. They start as round or irregular purple stains, which become elevated as smooth plaques after 3 to 4 weeks. If untreated, these plaques spread and become nodular before ulcerating. Lesions on the tongue are characteristically in the midline, and the thickness of the glossal epithelium hides the usual purple coloration. Small separate plaques on the gums are common, but in two patients we have seen the entire gingiva replaced by non-ulcerated nodular purple tissue, an event that is difficult to explain in terms of cancer growth.

The tonsils are often symmetrically enlarged but rarely show surface evidence of KS, and I have seen a plaque on the buccal mucosa only once.

I saw two patients in whom palatal plaques stopped at the edge of a dental plate, suggesting that steady pressure had inhibited spread. This, too, is difficult to explain if KS is indeed a sarcoma.

Oral lesions are satisfying to treat, since they disappear steadily and usually completely, retracing the stages by which they developed. Ulcers heal as nodularity diminishes; next smooth plaques flatten to form stains, which then fade to leave a stippling of pigment to mark their site.

Skin Lesions, Oedema and Infiltration

Skin lesions show a variety of appearances but are absent in about one-fifth of patients, who may, however, have diagnostic oral plaques. When present, skin lesions may be peripheral and nodular, as in endemic KS, but they are more often centrally located, on the face, neck, trunk or proximal parts of limbs: the typical form is a plaque. These are hyperpigmented, irregular in outline and often linear, following Langer's lines around the neck or on the back; they are raised from, and 1–2°C warmer than, surrounding skin. During rapid progression, a flare of purple discoloration may appear around pre-existing plaques, and this sign suggests a poor prognosis. Individual plaques are rarely larger than 3 cm in diameter, but in some sites, especially the medial aspects of both thighs, they are often multiple and confluent. Confluent plaques may become nodular and finally ulcerate, exuding offensive serous fluid in large amounts.

Plaques have a remarkably symmetrical distribution, particularly on the face, where the tip of the nose is the favourite site, but both cheeks and a U-shaped strip of skin around the pinna are also often involved. Plaques have been seen on the scalp if hair is sparse, but they are rare at this site. On the feet, plaques or infiltration are very common on the instep or under the toes but are almost unknown on the weightbearing surface of the sole; as usual, their distribution is symmetrical.

During treatment, ulcerated skin lesions cease to exude fluid and later epithelialize; next they flatten to form plaques, then stains or patches, and finally they disappear. They do so less rapidly than oral plaques and from above downwards, starting from the face (a happy chance for the patient, since embarrassingly visible lesions go first) and ending with the feet which is inexplicable as a manifestation of cancer responding to therapy.

Oedema occurs on the face, trunk or in a bikini distribution in about one-fifth of patients and suggests a poor prognosis, since 10 of 20 patients with this sign died at a median of 2 months from diagnosis (Bayley, 1988). Oedema has strange distributions; for example, it is common to find both legs oedematous to the groin except for the feet, or oedema may cover masses of enlarged nodes in both groins, yet the genitalia are not oedematous—observations that would seem to exclude central lymphatic obstruction as the cause of the oedema.

Infiltration is the term used to describe a woody induration of subcutaneous tissues that usually feel hot and fail to pit on pressure. It accompanies KS in both endemic and HIV related types but is more frequent in the former. The infiltration is common and symmetrical around confluent plaques on the medial thighs and groins. I have seen infiltration of the axillae and adjacent skin in only one patient (Fig. 2).

Pleural Effusions and Pulmonary Infiltration

Pleural effusions were seen, but very rarely, during proximal spread of infiltration to the trunk in men with endemic KS who had had symptoms for many years. Effusions are more common in patients with HIV related KS, but the most frequent radiological sign of pulmonary disease is infiltration of the lung

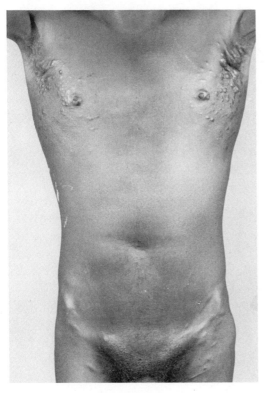

Fig. 2. Symmetrical infiltration around plaques in groin and axilla

parenchyma, which has never been described in endemic KS. It was first seen in 1983 when 4 of 13 patients presented with respiratory distress; in a later survey, 42% of new patients had clinical or radiological evidence of pulmonary disease, a larger proportion than would be seen in the West (Bayley, 1988). Symptoms start wth a dry cough, followed within 4 weeks by streak haemoptyses and dyspnoea, which worsens until some patients are bedridden. Clinical examination shows no abnormality at first, but later air entry to the lung bases is diminished and fine crepitations appear that do not clear on coughing. Serial chest radiographs show first a streaky appearance due to thickening of bronchovascular structures, followed by nearly symmetrical fluffy infiltrate radiating outwards from the hila of the lungs into the lower zones, but sparing the apices. The infiltrate extends in parallel with worsening dyspnoea.

The radiological changes (Fig. 3) resemble pulmonary oedema or lymphatic spread of carcinoma of the breast into the lungs. Miliary tuberculosis is more uniformly distributed across the whole lung field and opacities are denser and smaller.

Some patients with pulmonary KS are febrile, and many receive treatment for pulmonary tuberculosis even though their sputum does not show acid and alcohol fast bacilli. When symptoms and radiological signs fail to resolve, the diagnosis is questioned; examination of the mouth often reveals the true diagnosis.

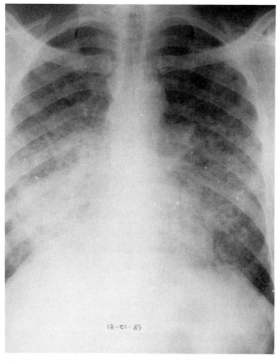

Fig. 3. Radiograph showing diffuse pulmonary changes

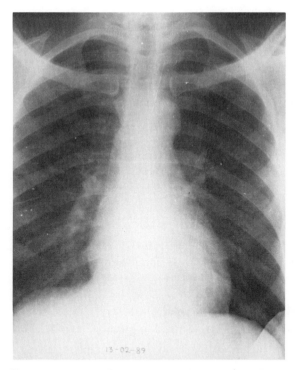

Fig. 4. Radiograph from the same patient after 1 month's treatment showing resolution of the lesions

Treatment with vincristine and either actinomycin D or epirubicin helps all but the most severely dyspnoeic patients, at least for a time, and is accompanied by partial or complete resolution of radiological changes (Fig. 4).

If treatment lapses completely, most patients have a recurrence of respiratory symptoms and signs about 4 months after their last dose of chemotherapy, although many respond a second time to the same agents. Pulmonary infiltration is the most common form of disease progression and also the most common immediate cause of death from HIV related KS in Zambia.

Opportunistic Infections

In Lusaka, unlike in the West, opportunistic infections do not dominate the clinical picture in patients with HIV related KS, and KS tends to behave more aggressively. The most common opportunist infections at presentation are candida and oral hairy leukoplakia; tuberculosis is suspected in some patients but is rarely proven.

During observation or treatment, the most common problem is pneumonia, which is suspected when the patient complains of sudden worsening of cough with lateral chest pain, fever and anorexia. Such episodes usually respond to antibiotics (erythromycin is particularly effective in my experience)

and do not interrupt therapy for more than 2 weeks. *Pneumocystis carinii* pneumonia is very rare in Zambia and Uganda, although it has been reported in Zimbabwe.

In the 5 year survey (Bayley, 1988) 13% of patients with KS had central nervous system signs at presentation, and 42% of these died at a median of less than 1 month, so encephalopathy is associated with a poor prognosis.

Is HIV Related Kaposi's Sarcoma a True Sarcoma?

HIV related KS does not behave like a malignant tumour (see Bayley and Lucas, 1990, for a fuller discussion). At presentation, most patients have multiple lesions that have developed rapidly and simultaneously in several different tissues, usually over a short space of time. Lesions show an inexplicable symmetry, and the distribution suggests that physical factors, including pressure and temperature, have influenced their positions. Treatment with cytotoxic drugs results in disappearance of many lesions by a process that seems to retrace the steps by which they developed, and disease in the mouth or on the head and neck fades first, together with pulmonary infiltration.

No malignant tumour (not excepting Burkitt's lymphoma) can grow so quickly, and no malignant tumour has a multicentric origin in cells of a single type distributed throughout the body in tissues as different as skin, lymph nodes, bronchus and oral epithelium. Moreover, malignant tumours usually start as a circumscribed nest of clearly abnormal cells at a single site where atypical or dysplastic cells are recognizable. In contrast, HIV related KS is difficult to detect in the early patch stage; the first histological change is the appearance of new structures (a fine network of capillaries) formed in the dermis (or the capsule of a lymph node or in lung septa) from apparently normal endothelial cells which show neither morphological changes nor an increased mitotic rate (Brooks, 1986; Cockerell, this issue).

There are even grounds for wondering whether KS tissue is able to exert an inhibitory effect on the replication or spread of HIV in the body. Life table curves show a curious tail of long term survivors from about 2 years after diagnosis. These survivors are not ill but well, in full time employment, muscular, well nourished and active.

MANAGEMENT

Diagnosis and Investigation

In most cases, a confident clinical diagnosis of HIV related KS can be made on inspection, because the multiple oral or skin lesions are unmistakable. Occasionally, red patches on the palate are difficult to interpret, but re-examination after an interval of 2 to 3 weeks nearly always removes doubt, since KS lesions enlarge and become raised during this period, while erythematous candida progresses to the membraneous stage. Biopsy is required to make a diagnosis of KS restricted to lymph nodes, but unless the nodes are large enough to cause discomfort or asymmetrical enough to raise the suspicion of tuberculosis or lymphoma, tissue diagnosis is not urgent or of real benefit to the patient. Biopsy is rarely necessary or desirable for the diagnosis of HIV related KS.

The extent or stage of disease influences prognosis and the choice of treatment. Careful clinical examination is the most important step, but a chest radiograph is needed to recognize early pulmonary infiltration, unexpected cavitating tuberculosis or a pericardial effusion (which may be due to KS but is more likely to be due to tuberculous pericarditis). A full blood count is essential to detect low platelet or granulocyte counts before treatment with cytotoxic drugs, and if a potentially cardiotoxic anthracycline is to be used, an electrocardiogram is desirable. No other investigations are relevant to management unless there are clinical signs of infection that demand special tests.

With the number of patients increasing, it is important to organize clinics efficiently to promote courteous reception of newcomers and the speedy completion of essential investigations. In Lusaka, new patients arrive early on the morning of a clinic day, to be greeted by experienced nurse-counsellors. New files are opened, patients are registered and then weighed and measured (for body surface area). A trained nurse or clinical officer counsels all patients, assesses their knowledge of HIV infection and AIDS and corrects important misconceptions. Patients are warned that HIV infection is one possible explanation for their symptoms, and they are asked whether they are willing to be tested and to hear their results later; very few refuse. Blood is drawn by venepuncture for a full blood count and for testing for antibodies to HIV. Finally, a standard history is taken, and the patient is sent for a chest radiograph and an electrocardiogram. Meanwhile, a full blood count is done, so that by the afternoon a clinic doctor has all the information needed to start treatment immediately if the patient agrees. Most patients are treated as outpatients, although a few (with respiratory distress, severe oedema or malnutrition) need admission for a few days at the start of therapy.

Prognostic Factors and Staging

In 1988, I compared the outcome of disease and the effects of treatment for groups of patients (from a consecutive series of 196 seen over a 5 year period) who had in common a single physical sign, for example, gross weight loss or oedema, recording median survival times for those who had died. In this way, I identified signs that were associated with death at a median of less than 2 months for 40% or more of a group. These were: weight loss in excess of 10 kg; clinical or radiographic evidence of respiratory tract disease; oedema of the head, trunk or bikini area; and central nervous system signs. The last sign was eliminated because it was probably not directly related to KS; a tentative staging scheme was developed from the remaining prognostic signs (Bayley, 1988) (see Table 1).

When patients were staged retrospectively with this scheme, life table curves were obtained for stage II and stage III that were clearly separated and yielded median survival times of greater than 3 years and 7.5 months, respectively. Experience over the next 3 years has confirmed the usefulness of this scheme with many more patients.

To Treat or Not to Treat?

When I saw patients with atypical KS for the first time in 1983, I treated them with the same drugs, actinomycin D and vincristine, that had proven value for endemic disease. Over half of these patients showed an excellent initial response, although this usually lasted for only 3 to 4 months in those who had stage III prognostic signs. Against this background, and with accumulating experience of rapid disease progression in the untreated, I did not consider a trial of chemotherapy versus no therapy ethically justifiable, so I offered treatment to all patients except stage I patients without symptoms.

In Lusaka, it is rare to see patients who have stage II disease that is neither disabling nor rapidly progressive, but in such circumstances I discuss the diagnosis with the patient, and we agree on a policy of observation or intravenous administration of vincristine as a single agent every 4 to 6 weeks. Radiotherapy in not available in Zambia or Uganda, although there are overstretched facilities in Kenya and Zimbabwe.

Clinicians with experience of HIV related KS in Europe or the USA who visit Africa comment that the disease tends to progress more rapidly and the proportion of patients who have pulmonary signs at presentation (42%) is higher than in the West. Zambian patients rarely have life threatening opportunistic infections at diagnosis, and KS is their chief problem, so after 7 years' experience I still cannot justify starting a study with a "no treatment" arm for those with advancing stage II or stage III disease.

TABLE 1. Staging of HIV related Kaposi's sarcoma

Stage I:	biopsy proven disease of lymph nodes, but no oral or skin lesions, no weight loss and a normal chest radiograph
Stage II:	any combination of lymph node, oral and skin disease, without (central) oedema of head, trunk or bikini area, with weight loss of less than 10 kg and a normal chest radiograph
Stage III:	oral, skin or node disease with weight loss in excess of 10 kg, and/or cough and dyspnoea accompanied by pulmonary infiltration or pleural effusion on a chest radiograph, and/or central oedema of head, trunk or bikini area

Actinomycin D and Vincristine

These drugs, given together, induced regression of endemic KS in around 90% of patients in Uganda (Olweny, 1981) and in 87% of patients treated in Lusaka (Bayley, 1988), although it is rare for signs to disappear totally. Disease often becomes active again after 1 to 2 years but nearly always responds promptly to the same treatment as before, usually for two or three recurrences. Over a period of 8 to 10 years, disease may become either less aggressive or (sometimes quite suddenly) much more aggressive, with rapid spread proximally and to the trunk.

The overall response rate to actinomycin D and vincristine for patients with HIV related KS is 61% but it rises to over 80% in those who have more than one course of treatment. It is not necessary to give daily actinomycin D or to give doses that would be used for cancer treatment, since a bolus dose of 1.5 to 2.0 mg (for an average adult) given with 2.0 mg vincristine every 3 to 4 weeks is effective, and regression has followed doses as low as 1.0 mg. It is difficult to control treatment induced vomiting and anorexia with the anti-emetics at our disposal, and many patients decline actinomycin D after the first one or two doses, especially if these are highly effective. For example, in a controlled trial of actinomycin D in comparison with epirubicin in Lusaka, all stage II patients having either treatment showed objective regressions at a second visit, but the median observation period for those receiving actinomycin D was 21 days, whereas for those receiving epirubicin it was 263 days (Bayley, 1990).

As in the management of endemic KS, reuse of the same therapy is often effective for more than one recurrence, but reactivation of disease occurs sooner with HIV related KS, at 4 or 5 months after the last course.

Phase II Trial of Epirubicin with Vincristine

Given the limited acceptance of actinomycin D and the ultimate failure of this drug to maintain control of HIV related KS, I sought an alternative treatment and chose epirubicin for a phase II trial in Lusaka. Experience in Uganda and Zambia had shown that adriamycin is active against both forms of KS, although it had never been tested in a formal trial. However, a less cardiotoxic anthracycline with a higher limiting dose was more attractive than the parent compound.

Patients with a clinical diagnosis of KS who were HIV positive and agreed to trial treatment were stratified as to stage and randomized within stages to receive either actinomycin D or epirubicin as a first treatment. Patients with disease confined to lymph nodes (stage I) were excluded. Both drugs were administered with vincristine at intervals of 21 or more days depending on blood counts.

We treated 69 men and 12 women in 1989 and early 1990. The overall sex ratio of 5.7:1 (M:F) concealed an uneven distribution of women, since half of

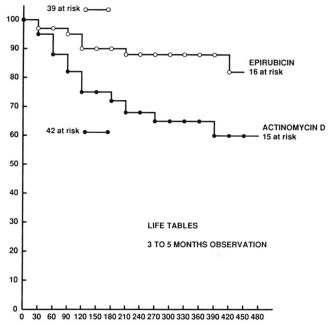

Fig. 5. Life table curves for KS patients treated with actinomycin D or epirubicin combined with vincristine

the women were in stage II (sex ratio 2.5:1); the sex ratio for stage III was 9:1 (M:F). Twenty one patients (26%) were in stage II and 60 (74%) in stage III.

All stage II patients and 73% of those in stage III showed objective disease regression after receiving epirubicin, while all stage II patients and 71% of those in stage III responded to actinomycin D. One stage II patient who received actinomycin D as first treatment died at 269 days after transfer to epirubicin on disease progression, but no stage II patients who received epirubicin as their first treatment are known to have died. In stage III, 10 of 31 patients who received actinomycin D were lost to follow-up, and 11 died at a median of 71 days from the start of therapy. Also in stage III, 6 of 29 patients who received epirubicin were lost to follow-up, and five died at a median of 73 days from the start of therapy. Figure 5 shows life table curves for all patients given each treatment, since the numbers were too small for separate analysis by stage. The difference between the curves is significant (p=0.04).

The most serious toxicity of epirubicin was onset of diarrhoea the week following therapy or exacerbation of pre-existing diarrhoea. Two patients died as a consequence of dehydration while their KS was regressing, so I no longer give epirubicin to anyone in whom diarrhoea cannot be controlled completely. No cardiotoxicity was seen, and a single death on the day of treatment (occurring in a patient who had received epirubicin) was thought to be disease rather than drug related. Two patients who had excellent disease regression had outbreaks of maculopapular dermatosis on two or more occasions about 5 days after administration of epirubicin, and itching and ulceration were so severe that epirubicin had to be discontinued. These were the only patients transferred to treatment with actinomycin D, whereas 11 were transferred to epirubicin because progressing disease failed to respond to retreatment with actinomycin D.

In conclusion, HIV related KS regressed in response to epirubicin, and this drug was preferred by patients. Uncontrolled diarrhoea contraindicated its use, but otherwise epirubicin was associated with increased survival times (Bayley, 1990) and was particularly useful in stage II patients.

In the phase II trial of epirubicin, a dose of 90 mg/m^2 was used, repeated every 21 days if marrow toxicity permitted. However, at the end of the trial, as continuing regression had been observed in patients who had infrequent treatment or reduced doses on account of low platelet or granulocyte counts, we began to give lower doses to conserve waning supplies of epirubicin. Our pilot experience suggests that a dose of 60 mg/m^2 is effective, and a formal trial at this dose level (or less frequent administration of standard doses) would be worthwhile.

A maintenance treatment to postpone reactivation of disease following the end of chemotherapy would be useful, particularly for stage III patients. When treatment is stopped, renewed disease activity is seen after 4 months (unpublished observations) in 66% of patients who attended for follow-up, usually as cough and dyspnoea due to pulmonary infiltration. Vincristine at a dose of 2.0 mg every 6 to 8 weeks was given to a few patients for periods of up to 2 years without recurrence of disease activity or neurological toxicity, so this drug would be worth a formal trial as a maintenance therapy.

Adjuncts to Chemotherapy

Physical treatments may be useful as adjuncts to chemotherapy. For example, steady application of pressure to suitably sited skin lesions (using pressure garments of the type used to prevent or treat keloids) might hasten regression of slowly responding plaques on limbs or prevent their reappearance. Similarly, the local application of heat might be investigated, since the distribution of skin lesions suggests that they develop most easily at cool sites (tip of nose, cheeks, feet). Finally, the disappearance of plaques from above downwards during drug therapy suggests that simple elevation (to improve venous and lymphatic drainage) could be tried in the management of obstinate lower limb lesions, but only as an adjunct to drugs.

Patients who remain well and active 2 or more years after diagnosis (especially if they had stage III signs at presentation) form a group needing detailed study to investigate the interaction of HIV and KS. Serial counts of CD4 and CD8 positive lymphocytes, with serial isolation and characterization of HIV from peripheral blood cells, may suggest the mechanism by which health is being maintained and could encourage trial of small doses of cytotoxic drugs in the management of HIV related pathologies other than Kaposi's "sarcoma."

For example, thrombocytopaenia is a common complication of HIV infection and may be troublesome at an early stage when patients are otherwise in good health. In Lusaka, we have treated thrombocytopaenia occurring in KS with intravenous vincristine at a dose of 2.0 mg with consistently good results. (On two occasions, patients were bleeding actively, and, to our surprise, bleeding ceased within a few hours of treatment.) Platelet levels rise to normal and regression of KS begins, preparing the way for treatment with myelotoxic drugs later. We do not know the mechanism by which platelet production and activity are restored, but it is a useful effect and deserves study; intermittent administration of vincristine would seem to be preferable to splenectomy in already immunocompromised patients, regardless of whether or not they have KS.

Decentralization of Management to District Hospitals

In Lusaka, the number of new patients with HIV related KS presenting at one clinic in a year rose from 14 in 1983 to 196 in 1989, and records suggest a new patient enrollment of over 300 persons by the end of 1990. Moreover, lymph node biopsies indicate that KS develops in about 10% of HIV positive adults at some time, at least in Zambia. These figures imply that in African countries with a type 2 epidemic, large numbers of new patients with a treatable consequence of HIV infection will present each year for at least the next 2 decades. It is unrealistic to expect them to be treated at a central hospital, and it would be inhumane to withhold cost effective therapy that could allow many persons to function normally at work and at home. In these circumstances, we need standard treatment schedules that can be managed safely by district hospital doctors or clinical officers and an organization similar to the tuberculosis treatment service to supervise and encourage them.

In Zambia, a 3 day seminar was held in 1990 to teach district hospital doctors and clinical officers to recognize and manage KS. We handed out detailed lecture notes, showed many colour slides and provided several opportunities for participants to examine patients and to discuss their management. At the conclusion of the course, doctors were provided with supplies of cytotoxic drugs to take back to their stations for immediate use, and we plan to maintain drug supplies through provincial medical officers while collecting basic information about numbers of patients treated and the results of therapy for a central register. After a year, a follow-up workshop of briefer duration will be held. All participants were urged to teach other doctors or clinical officers in their own and nearby hospitals what they had learned, and in this way we hope that knowledge about KS will spread throughout the country. Standards of care for individual patients may decline at first, but larger numbers should be recognized and treated. A decentralized treatment service should be supported by a strong but small central referral clinic from which trial work can be done and refresher courses organized and where research records can be collected and analyzed.

Effects on the Family and Care in the Home

Many patients with KS do not want to tell their partners that they are HIV infected, so we are not able to test the partners for antibodies, but evidence from a sexually transmitted diseases clinic suggests that at least 60% of spouses are or become HIV positive. In two instances, KS developed in the second partner, but other HIV related pathologies are much more common. I ask about the health of the spouse and youngest child at all first visits and at intervals thereafter and encourage the index patient to bring sick relatives to the clinic.

It is realistic to expect most stage II and some stage III patients to return to work, and I resist pressure to agree to retirement on medical grounds until I am sure that this is inevitable. I encourage patients to hope for long term control of symptoms with (perhaps) some residual disability and teach an assertive attitude to both KS and HIV. The patient is the chief protagonist and should not be relegated to a passive role in the team; he or she can and will learn a good deal about drug effects and disease behaviour (and patient's observations may provide clues to the alert researcher), but patients do tend to underestimate regression in response to therapy. It is vital that the clinician maintains a hopeful and fighting spirit, even when the goal of treatment must shift from disease control to symptom control during the terminal phase of the illness.

In Lusaka, we started a homecare service in 1987 to keep patients at home with their families and reduce the costs of care, to release hospital beds for patients with acute treatable disease that is not HIV related and to enhance the impact of education programmes by keeping the consequences of infection visible in the community. Families provide no less effective care than hospitals, given a little support and simple drug supplies, and if wards are crowded and staff morale is poor, care in the home is likely to be of higher quality.

CONCLUSIONS

1. Like all HIV related disease, KS is a family problem in Africa.
2. Management can and should be based in clinics and in the home.
3. As KS develops in a large proportion of HIV infected persons in Africa, national treatment programmes are needed (analogous to programmes for management of tuberculosis) using standard treatment schemes and trained district doctors or paramedical staff.
4. Most patients show disease regression after treatment with cytotoxic drugs, and at least a quarter have a median survival time in excess of 3 years. Treatment is cost effective and can be standardized.
5. HIV related KS does not behave like a typical malignant tumour. We should test the hypothesis that it results from proliferation of untransformed endothelium (in response to systemic and local growth factors).

SUMMARY

The incidence of HIV related KS has increased 50-fold since it was first recognized in Zambia in 1983. The mean age at diagnosis is 35 years for men and 28 years for women, with a sex ratio of M:F=5:1. The most common symptoms and signs are weight loss, symmetrical lymphadenopathy, oral plaques, skin plaques in a central distribution, oedema and cough with dyspnoea. Biopsy is needed to confirm the diagnosis if disease is confined to lymph nodes. Objective regression occurs in 80% of patients receiving adequate doses of actinomycin D and vincristine (median survival time >3 years for stage I or II disease and 7.5 months for stage III); epirubicin with vincristine was more effective in a phase II trial. Both treatments give good relief of symptoms, allowing patients to return to work.

Clinical, histological and biological features of HIV related KS do not support conclusively its classification as a "malignant tumour".

Heterosexual and perinatal transmission of HIV in Africa ensures that KS affects families, not just individuals.

Acknowledgements

I am grateful for the hard work and compassion of the staff who work in the Tumour Clinic at the University Teaching Hospital in Lusaka, and particularly Mr Juston Daka, who guards records. Without the courage and confidence of hundreds of Zambian men and women with Kaposi's disease none of this work could have been done: they are my friends and I salute them. I thank the Medical Illustration Unit of the University Teaching Hospital, Lusaka, for the illustrations, and Dr Limbambala, Executive Director of that Hospital, for his support. The World Health Organization provided funds for the 1990 short course on Kaposi's disease for district doctors and clinical officers, and I am grateful to Dr Eric van Praag, WHO teamleader in Lusaka, who encouraged me to decentralize care. I also thank Farmitalia for a generous donation of epirubicin for the phase II trial.

References

Ackerman LV and Murray JF (1962) *Symposium on Kaposi's Sarcoma, Union Internationalis Contra Cancrum.* Karger, Basel

Bayley AC (1984) Aggressive Kaposi's sarcoma in Zambia: 1983. *Lancet* **i** 1318

Bayley AC, Cheingsong-Popov R, Dalgleish AG, Downing RG, Tedder RS and Weiss RA (1985) HTLV III serology distinguishes atypical and endemic Kaposi's sarcoma in Africa. *Lancet* **i** 359–361

Bayley AC (1988) Atypical African Kaposi's sarcoma, In: Giraldo G, Beth-Giraldo E, Clumeck N, Gharbi Md-R, Kyalwazi SK and de Thé G (eds). *AIDS and Associated Cancers in Africa*, pp 152–164, Karger, Basel

Bayley AC (1990) Epirubicin is active against African HIV-related Kaposi's sarcoma. Sixth International Conference on AIDS, June 1990 [Abstract SB 25]

Bayley AC and Lucas SB (1990) Kaposi's sarcoma or Kaposi's disease? In: Fletcher CDM and

McKee PH (eds). *Current Problems in Tumour Pathology: Pathobiology of Soft Tissue Tumours,* pp 141–163, Churchill Livingstone, Edinburgh

Brooks JJ (1986) Kaposi's sarcoma: a reversible hyperplasia. *Lancet* **ii** 1309–1311

Hutt MSR (1981) Pathology of Kaposi's sarcoma, In: Olweny CLM, Hutt MSR and Owor R (eds). *Antibiotics and Chemotherapy,* vol 29, pp 32–37, Karger, Basel

Khorshid KA, Erzingatzian K, Watters DAK and Bayley AC (1987) Intussusception due to Kaposi's sarcoma. *Journal of the Royal College of Surgeons of Edinburgh* **32** 339–341

Olweny CLM (1981) Management of Kaposi's sarcoma. Chemotherapy II, In: Olweny CLM, Hutt MSR and Owor R (eds). *Antibiotics and Chemotherapy,* vol 29, pp 88–95, Karger, Basel

Vogel CL (1981) Management of Kaposi's sarcoma. Chemotherapy I, In: Olweny CLM, Hutt MSR and Owor R (eds). *Antibiotics and Chemotherapy,* vol 29, pp 82–87, Karger, Basel

Watters DAK, Sinclair JR, Luo N and Verma R (1988) HIV seroprevalence in critically ill patients in Zambia. *AIDS* **2** 142–143

The author is responsible for the accuracy of the references.

Histopathological Features of Kaposi's Sarcoma in HIV Infected Individuals

C J COCKERELL

The University of Texas Southwestern Medical School, 5323 Harry Hines Blvd, Dallas, Texas 75235-9072

Introduction
    Frequency and prevalence of Kaposi's sarcoma
    Importance of accurate diagnosis of Kaposi's sarcoma
    Biopsy technique
Histological development of Kaposi's sarcoma from patch to tumour types
    Diffuse vascular proliferation
    Patch stage disease
    Plaque stage disease
    Nodules and tumours
Histological variants
    Angiomatous form
    Traumatized lesions
    Coexisting Kaposi's sarcoma and bacillary angiomatosis
    Resolving lesions
    Extracutaneous Kaposi's sarcoma
Histological simulators of Kaposi's sarcoma
    Angioma
    Bacillary angiomatosis
    Acroangiodermatitis
    Angiosarcomata
    Spindle cell neoplasms
    Inflammatory dermatoses
    Dermatofibroma and scar
    Miscellaneous conditions
Additional points
Conclusion
Summary

INTRODUCTION

Frequency and Prevalence of Kaposi's Sarcoma

Kaposi's sarcoma (KS) is the neoplasm most commonly found in patients infected with HIV. Although the frequency of KS has been declining (Drew *et al*, 1988) up to 35% of homosexual men may develop KS at some point during their disease (Longo *et al*, 1984) and at necropsy, up to 95% of all patients with AIDS have been shown to have either cutaneous or visceral KS (Niedt and Schinella, 1985). This neoplasm is responsible for extensive morbidity in these individuals and may be associated with increased mortality.

Importance of Accurate Diagnosis of Kaposi's Sarcoma

It is important that KS is recognized and diagnosed with certainty for a number of reasons. Firstly, the development of KS is an AIDS defining event (Centers for Disease Control, 1985). Although original studies in the mid 1980s indicated that patients who presented with KS had a better long term prognosis than those who presented with an opportunistic infection (Chachoua *et al*, 1989) these demographic findings have changed somewhat in the past few years because of more careful monitoring and early administration of prophylactic antibiotics. In addition, the development of AIDS associated KS is associated with diminished CD4 cell numbers and lowered CD4:CD8 ratios (Taylor *et al*, 1986). Furthermore, KS may be the presenting sign of HIV infection. It is not uncommon that a biopsy specimen submitted as an angioma or other benign vascular lesion in a patient not thought to have HIV infection is subsequently shown to be KS associated with AIDS. Finally, some conditions may be confused with KS both clinically and histologically. Many of these may have serious consequences if left untreated.

It is especially important that histopathologists are aware of the numerous forms KS shows, both in the skin and in visceral organs. Failure to recognize KS histologically may lead to patients going undiagnosed and untreated, leaving them vulnerable to opportunistic infections. Overdiagnosis may lead to anxiety, severe psychological problems and suicide.

In general, KS in HIV infected individuals has histological features similar to those of classical KS seen in elderly individuals. Clinically, as mentioned elsewhere in this chapter, the two conditions are quite distinct in their distribution, rapidity of spread and response to treatment. HIV associated KS is similar both to KS that arises in other immunocompromised patients and to the epidemic African form of KS.

Biopsy Technique

To arrive at a precise histopathological diagnosis of KS, it is important that an adequate biopsy of a lesion be performed. Because this neoplasm presents most commonly in the skin, punch or incisional biopsies are preferred methods of sampling KS lesions. Kaposi's sarcoma, especially in early stages, tends to involve the reticular dermis more than the superficial papillary dermis; thus a superficial biopsy may merely fail to be deep enough for a precise diagnosis to be made. In addition, on occasion, lesions may be associated with other vascular proliferations such as pyogenic granuloma, and a superficial biopsy may sample an area of granulation tissue rather than the neoplastic process.

In this chapter, the histopathological findings of KS in the skin of HIV infected individuals will be addressed, with emphasis on cutaneous lesions. The chronological evolution of KS will be dealt with first, followed by a discussion of variants of KS and finally, histological simulators.

HISTOLOGICAL DEVELOPMENT OF KAPOSI'S SARCOMA FROM PATCH TO TUMOUR TYPES

Diffuse Vascular Proliferation

The very earliest histological change of KS may not represent KS at all. One study has demonstrated a subtle proliferation of blood vessels in clinically unaffected skin of individuals with AIDS, a finding that may be the earliest manifestation of impending KS (Ruszczak *et al*, 1987). This may be a consequence of either a generalized viral infection involving endothelial cells in widespread fashion (Dictor and Jarplid, 1988) or the effect of some circulating vascular proliferation factor (Salahuddin *et al*, 1988). Such changes may be extremely subtle and difficult to interpret histologically even in those such as homosexual men in whom the incidence of KS is quite high. In many cases the vascular proliferation may not be present at all; furthermore, in patients with well developed KS, biopsies of skin taken for other reasons usually fail to reveal vascular proliferation. Nevertheless, we have experience with a number of biopsy specimens from patients with HIV infection and KS that did show proliferations of vessels that could not be diagnosed as KS.

Patch Stage Disease

The earliest recognizable form of KS is early "patch stage" disease (Figs. 1–5). Clinically, skin lesions are usually characterized by small pinkish macules that can be difficult to recognize as KS. In general, two histological patterns of patch stage KS have been described (Ackerman, 1979; Gottleib and Ackerman, 1988). In one type, there is an increased number of dilated vascular spaces, with irregular shapes, lined by thin, flattened endothelial cells. The vascular spaces are often difficult to appreciate, but when present, they appear to dissect between collagen bundles in the upper reticular dermis. Characteristically in this form of patch stage KS, pre-existing blood vessels and adnexal structures are surrounded by a vascular proliferation that may appear to protrude into vascular lumina. This has been referred to as the "promontory" sign (Fig. 3). There is also an infiltrate of lymphocytes and plasma cells interstitially between vessels, associated with extravasated erythrocytes and siderophages. The endothelial cells lining the bizarre blood vessels are either thin and spindle shaped or somewhat oval or round. Most of the endothelial cells are without evidence of mitoses or pleomorphism (Ackerman, 1979; Gottleib and Ackerman, 1988).

The second pattern of patch stage KS consists of a proliferation of spindle and oval endothelial cells almost exclusively around pre-existing blood vessels of the upper reticular dermis. This has been referred to as "pseudo-granulomatous" because the aggregations of plump endothelial cells surrounded by plasma cells and lymphocytes give a histological appearance similar to a small granuloma. Small vascular spaces and extravasation of erythrocytes are also observed. In addition to these two patterns, there may be overlap with features of both in the same specimen. Features common to both patterns include the presence of clefts lined with thin endothelial cells between collagen bundles. This correlates with the electron microscopic finding of pseudopodia of endothelial cells extending for long distances along collagen bundles.

Plaque Stage Disease

In time, the vascular proliferation may become more extensive and spread to involve most of the reticular dermis as well as the upper subcutaneous fat. This more densely cellular variant of KS is clinically recognizable as either a papule or a plaque and histologically is referred to as the plaque stage (Figs. 6 and 7) (Lever and Schaumburg-Lever, 1983; Gottleib and Ackerman, 1988; Santucci et al, 1988). The tendency of the abnormal vessels to be mostly interstitial or mostly perivascular is maintained, but a greater number of endothelial cells in the lesion results in a caricature of the patch stage. Blood vessels are very bizarre and jagged but thin walled. Occasionally, rounded thick walled vessels may be seen admixed with the neoplastic vessels. Such vessels may represent pre-existing plexuses or abnormal vessels altered by stasis when lesions are in the lower extremities. The inflammatory cell infiltrate in plaque lesions is more dense, and sometimes small nodules of plasma cells are seen throughout the lesion. Extravasated erythrocytes and siderophages may be numerous. Because of the abundant extravasation of erythrocytes, erythrophagocytosis is often seen. The breakdown products of phagocytosed erythrocytes take on a pinkish refractile appearance. The structures have been referred to as "hyalin globules", and although they are not specific for KS, they are a helpful finding when the diagnosis is in question (Lever and Schaumburg-Lever, 1983; Gottleib and Ackerman, 1988; Santucci et al, 1988).

Nodules and Tumours

Finally, some lesions may progress to form nodules and tumours (Figs. 8 and 9). The nodular stage of KS is a spindle cell neoplastic process characterized by interweaving fascicles of spindle cells (Lever and Schaumburg-Lever, 1983; Gottleib and Ackerman, 1988; Santucci et al, 1988). Extravasated erythrocytes

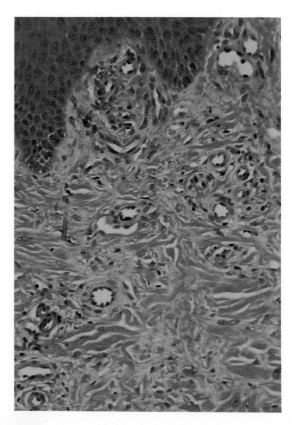

Fig. 1. Very early patch stage KS. There is an increase in the number of vascular spaces surrounding small plexuses of blood vessels in the upper reticular dermis. (Haematoxylin and eosin, magnification x7500)

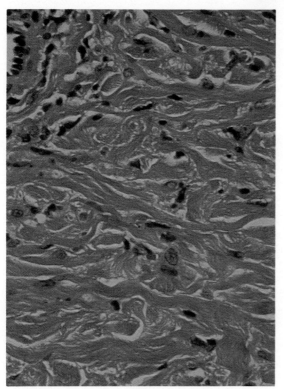

Fig. 2. Patch stage KS. Between collagen bundles in the dermis are an increased number of slit like vascular spaces lined by thin endothelial cells. (Haematoxylin and eosin, magnification, x120 000)

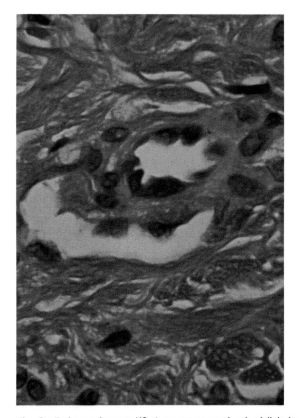

Fig. 3. Early patch stage KS. A promontory sign is visible here, namely, a pre-existing blood vessel appearing to protrude into the lumen of a newly formed neoplastic one. (Haematoxylin and eosin, magnification x186 000)

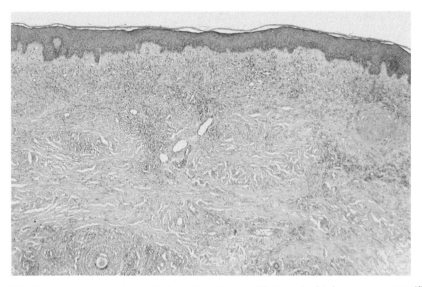

Fig. 4. More fully developed lesion of patch stage KS. Even in this low power magnification, the pattern is that of a proliferative perivascular process with numerous slits that represent vascular spaces. (Haematoxylin and eosin, magnification x4650)

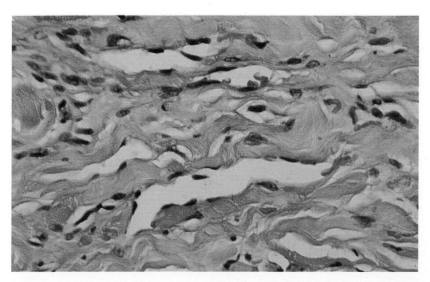

Fig. 5. Patch stage KS, more fully developed lesion. An increased number of jagged, bizarre vascular spaces are seen between collagen bundles in the dermis. Scattered extravasated erythrocytes and siderophages may also be present. Note the lining of the blood vessels by thin endothelial cells. (Haematoxylin and eosin, magnification x155 000)

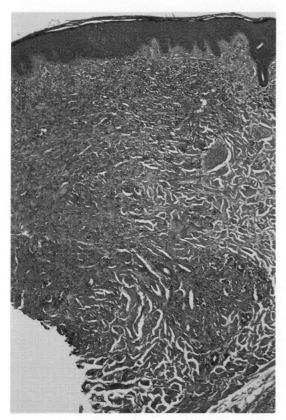

Fig. 6. Plaque stage KS. Note the more densely cellular and diffuse nature of the process. The numerous clefts are signs of vascular differentiation. (Haematoxylin and eosin, magnification x7750)

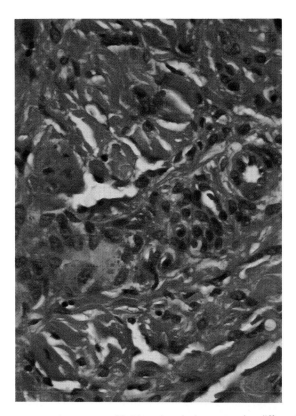

Fig. 7. Plaque stage KS. Note the obvious vascular differentiation with the neoplasm consisting of innumerable plump and spindle shaped endothelial cells. Note also the scattered extravasated erythrocytes and the pre-existing blood vessel around which the neoplastic process is situated. (Haematoxylin and eosin, magnification x124 000)

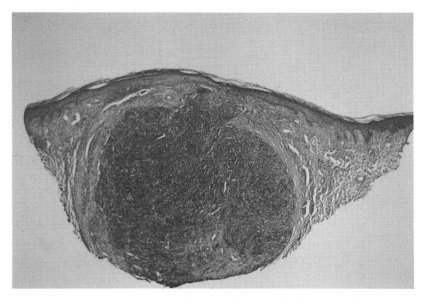

Fig. 8. Nodular stage KS. There is a densely cellular neoplastic process that extends from the reticular dermis to the subcutaneous fat. (Haematoxylin and eosin, magnification x3100)

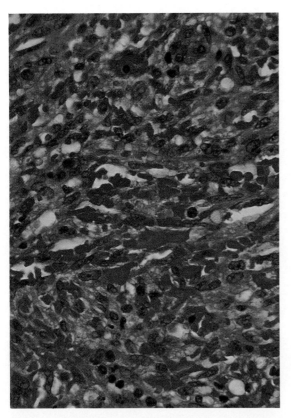

Fig. 9. KS, nodular type. There are fascicles of spindle cells comprising this neoplasm that interweave. Numerous extravasated erythrocytes are present as well as small round spaces that are attempts at vascular differentiation. Plasma cells and hyalin globules are found scattered throughout the lesion. (Haematoxylin and eosin, magnification x124 000)

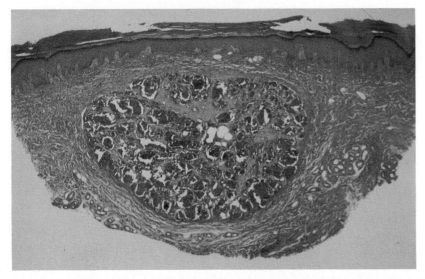

Fig. 10. Angiomatous type of KS. On low magnification there is a vascular process with numerous cavernous vascular spaces with an overall appearance similar to an angioma. (Haematoxylin and eosin, magnification x4650)

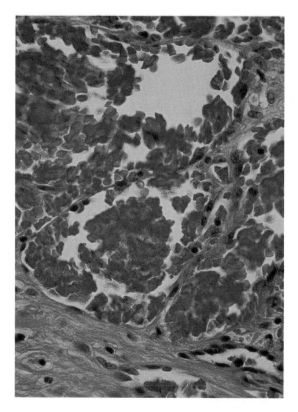

Fig. 11. Higher magnification reveals the vascular spaces to be somewhat irregular and lined by thin rather than plump endothelial cells. Although the spaces are filled with erythrocytes, no thrombosis is seen. (Haematoxylin and eosin, magnification x124 000)

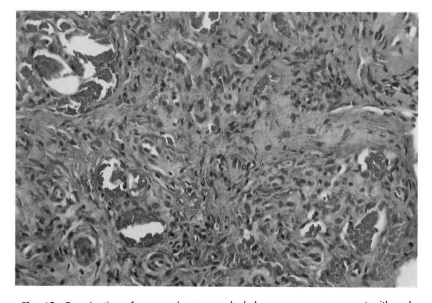

Fig. 12. Examination of a second area revealed changes more consonant with early nodular stage KS. Note the beginnings of fascicles of cells that interweave and blend perceptibly with the angiomatous areas. (Haematoxylin and eosin, magnification x77 500)

are abundant between individual spindle cells. Careful examination shows that small round spaces between individual fascicles of spindle cells represent vascular spaces. The progression from a plaque to a KS nodule is sometimes seen within the same specimen. Individual nodules may increase in size from a solitary focus, or large nodules and tumours may be the consequence of coalescence of smaller aggregations of spindle cells. The neoplastic cells characteristically have elongated nuclei with somewhat vesicular chromatin and vacuolation of the cytoplasm. Atypia is a prominent feature in these lesions, and numerous mitotic figures and striking pleomorphism are commonly observed. Nodules may be located at any site within the skin, with the reticular dermis being involved most commonly, but subcutaneous fat as well as the papillary dermis may be affected (Safai *et al*, 1985; Muggia and Lonberg, 1986). In some cases, the lesions may be quite deeply situated and may be connected to underlying fascia, muscle and even bone (Safai *et al*, 1985; Muggia and Lonberg, 1986). Occasionally, lesions may be pedunculated and surrounded by epithelial collars. Ulceration and zones of necrosis may be seen. Inflammatory infiltrates are predominantly lymphoplasmacytic, with other cells being present less frequently.

HISTOLOGICAL VARIANTS

Angiomatous Form

In addition to the KS types discussed above, there are a number of histological variants that may cause confusion in diagnosis. A not uncommon variant of KS is the so-called "angiomatous" form (Figs. 10 and 11) (Gottleib and Ackerman, 1988). In this lesion, there are well formed blood vessels that are somewhat irregular in size and shape and are usually aggregated. Vascular spaces are lined by thin, flattened endothelial cells rather than round or plump cells characteristically seen in angiomata. Such vascular spaces may be present in the mid dermis but can be associated with pre-existing adnexal structures or normal appearing blood vessels. In addition, it is not uncommon for the vascular spaces of angiomatous KS to be filled with erythrocytes. This should be distinguished from thrombosis, which is not an uncommon finding in normal angiomata after trauma. In addition, on occasion the red blood cells within the lumina of angiomatous lesions of KS may assume an orange colour. The reason for this is unclear. Despite these features, it may be quite difficult to distinguish an angiomatous KS lesion from a true angioma in some cases. As a general rule, careful evaluation of surrounding areas will reveal features of patch and/or plaque stage KS (Fig. 12) (Gottleib and Ackerman, 1988).

Traumatized Lesions

A KS lesion may be traumatized, resulting in a superimposed granulation tissue response. In such cases, superficial biopsy results for granulation tissue may be interpreted as either a pyogenic granuloma or as granulation tissue. It is important to be aware that this phenomenon can occur and to mention in the pathology report that the biopsy was taken superficially and that the stated diagnosis may be a consequence of a sampling error. Only when deeper biopsies are done will the more characteristic features of KS be seen.

Coexisting Kaposi's Sarcoma and Bacillary Angiomatosis

The same can be said of lesions of KS and bacillary epithelioid angiomatosis (BEA) occurring in contiguity (Berger *et al*, 1989). Bacillary epithelioid angiomatosis is characterized by a proliferation of round blood vessels with epithelioid endothelial cells, many of which protrude into vascular lumina (Cockerell and LeBoit, 1990). An inflammatory cell infiltrate of numerous neutrophils is characteristically seen, with scattered deposits of purplish granular material corresponding to colonies of bacteria. A Warthin-Starry stain of BEA reveals clumps of bacilli in the angiomatosis areas (Cockerell and LeBoit, 1990). No bacteria are seen in the KS areas.

Resolving Lesions

Kaposi's sarcoma lesions that have undergone resolution as a result of therapy with X irradiation, topical application of liquid nitrogen or chemotherapy may have features that are not diagnostic of KS. Histologically, one sees abundant siderophages, dermal fibroplasia and sclerosis and only scattered residual endothelial cells between collagen bundles. Soon after treatment, especially of nodules, there may be a dense inflammatory cell infiltrate with extensive necrosis of endothelial cells (Gottleib and Ackerman, 1988).

Extracutaneous Kaposi's Sarcoma

Extracutaneous KS may differ histologically and may have a slightly different developmental chronology than KS lesions in the skin. The most commonly affected sites other than the skin are the lymph nodes, the gastrointestinal tract and the respiratory tract (Niedt and Schinella, 1985). In lymph nodes, the earliest changes are those that have been referred to as "hypervascular follicular hyperplasia" (Lubin and Rywlin, 1971). Vascular channels within the node are prominent, increased in number and associated with an increase in the number of plasma cells (Amazon and Rywlin, 1979). In time, these areas may develop more classical findings of KS, namely, interweaving fascicles of spindle cells, vascular slits and extravasation of erythrocytes with siderophages. Entire lymph nodes may eventually be replaced with fully developed KS (Amazon and Rywlin, 1979, 1988).

The gastrointestinal tract is also commonly involved. Virtually the entire tract from the oral cavity to the anus may be affected (Amazon and Rywlin,

1988). In general, the histological findings are similar to those seen in the skin, although angiomatous features may be seen somewhat more commonly. Early lesions of KS may show dilated irregular blood vessels not easily recognizable as KS (Amazon and Rywlin, 1988). Similar findings have also been reported in early lesions of the pulmonary parenchyma (Amazon and Rywlin, 1988).

HISTOLOGICAL SIMULATORS OF KAPOSI'S SARCOMA

Kaposi's sarcoma may simulate a number of different processes in the skin, both inflammatory and neoplastic (Hennessey and Friedman-Kien, 1989). Conversely, KS may be simulated by a number of different entities. If the criteria outlined above are applied carefully, it is unlikely that confusion in diagnosis will result.

Angioma

Probably the most common simulator of KS is an angioma. Clinically, such lesions are vascular in appearance, and in patients at risk for HIV disease, KS will be the most likely clinical diagnosis. Histologically, angiomata are almost always associated with plump, round endothelial cells which line vascular lumina (Lever and Schaumburg-Lever, 1983; Gottleib and Ackerman, 1988). Such vessels may be located superficially without a tendency to involve deeper vessels such as the mid vascular plexus and usually have no tendency to be centred around pre-existing blood vessels or adnexal structures. Furthermore, the pattern of an angioma is usually homogeneous, whereas in a specific KS lesion, progression from patch to nodular stages may be seen (Gottleib and Ackerman, 1988).

Bacillary Angiomatosis

Bacillary epithelioid angiomatosis occasionally may be confused with KS, but, in my opinion, the two do not simulate one another histologically with great frequency. Bacillary epithelioid angiomatosis is characterized by a lobular proliferation of round blood vessels with thick, plump ("epithelioid") endothelial cells (Cockerell and LeBoit, 1990). Numerous neutrophils are commonly seen in densely cellular lesions, a finding almost never seen in KS. Finally, stains for bacteria would readily distinguish the two (Cockerell and LeBoit, 1990).

Acroangiodermatitis

Severe stasis changes, especially those that have evolved to acroangiodermatitis, may be confused clinically with KS (Hennessey and Friedman-Kien, 1989). Histologically, the lesion is readily distinguished from plaque stage KS because individual blood vessels are thick walled, round and lined with plump endothelial cells. No tendency to the formation of bizarre jagged blood vessels surrounding pre-existing ones is seen (Gottleib and Ackerman, 1988). When stasis changes are superimposed on lesions of KS, the vascular changes of stasis mentioned above are seen in the superficial portion of the specimen, with more characteristic features of patch and plaque stage KS seen beneath (Gottleib and Ackerman, 1988).

Angiosarcomata

Rarely, KS may simulate angiosarcomata and vice versa. In general, the endothelial cells lining the neoplastic vascular spaces of angiosarcoma are large and lined by endothelial cells that are strikingly pleomorphic and atypical. Aggregations of neoplastic endothelial cells may be present freely within lumina of vascular spaces, a finding not seen in KS (Lever and Schaumburg-Lever, 1983; Gottleib and Ackerman, 1988). Angiosarcomata are almost never lined by thin typical endothelial cells.

Spindle Cell Neoplasms

Other spindle cell neoplastic processes may mimic KS, especially if lesions are examined with high magnification. Kaposi's sarcoma lesions are almost always associated with vascular slits and usually contain numerous extravasated erythrocytes. Careful searches for signs of differentiation within other spindle cell neoplasms will usually aid in distinguishing them from KS. For example, the presence of melanin and evidence of cornification will distinguish spindle cell melanomas and spindle cell carcinomas from KS, respectively (Gottleib and Ackerman, 1988). Nevertheless, in some cases, the similarity between spindle cell neoplasms and KS may be so great as to require immunoperoxidase studies. Obviously, KS stains for vascular associated antigens such as factor VIII and *Ulex europaeus* (Lever and Schaumburg-Lever, 1983).

Inflammatory Dermatoses

Occasionally, inflammatory conditions may simulate KS. Granuloma annulare, especially the interstitial form, may be associated with perivascular infiltrates of epithelioid cells and lymphocytes simulating a patch stage lesion of KS with a "pseudogranulomatous" appearance (Gottleib and Ackerman, 1988). Careful evaluation reveals that the epithelioid cells represent histiocytes, and the absence of plasma cells in the infiltrate is another clue that such a lesion is not KS. Necrobiosis lipoidica may simulate patch stage lesions of KS, but the degree of sclerosis and the presence of fibrin within the centres of areas of palisaded granulomatous inflammation are not characteristic of KS (Gottleib and Ackerman, 1988). Finally, early patch stage KS lesions may simulate persistent purpuric dermatitis (Gottleib and Ackerman, 1988). Careful evaluation of such lesions will reveal the vascular spaces lined by the thin endothelial cells.

Dermatofibroma and Scar

Finally, fibroblastic proliferations such as dermatofibromata and scars may either simulate KS or be simulated by it (Gottleib and Ackerman, 1988). Once again, inspection of the vessels within a dermatofibroma reveals them to be round and thick walled and associated with an inflammatory infiltrate of histiocytes, many of which may be multinucleated. The characteristic change of epidermal hyperplasia overlying a dermatofibroma is yet another clue to the diagnosis. Scars may be associated with a vascular proliferation that usually consists of round endothelial cells. Such vascular proliferations in scars are also associated with abundant, newly formed basophilic collagen.

Miscellaneous Conditions

Other conditions that have been reported occasionally to mimic KS include pyogenic granuloma, spindle and epithelioid cell naevus (Spitz's naevus) and pseudolymphoma.

ADDITIONAL POINTS

Although the development of KS in patients at risk of HIV disease is currently thought to be an AIDS defining event, recent evidence indicates that KS may occur in individuals who do not have HIV infection but have risk factors for the infection (Friedman-Kien et al, 1990). Kaposi's sarcoma in such patients has a clinical appearance similar to classical KS. The recognition of this phenomenon has raised speculation that KS may be caused by a virus unrelated to HIV (Dictor and Jarplid, 1988). Indeed, virus particles shown to be morphologically dissimilar to HIV have been demonstrated in KS lesions, both classical and AIDS associated (Barbanti-Brodano et al, 1987; McDougall et al, 1987; Grody et al, 1988; Rappersberger et al, 1990). It is anticipated that the aetiological agent will be identified soon.

CONCLUSION

Kaposi's sarcoma, the most common and most important cutaneous neoplasm in patients with HIV disease, may be readily recognized by its pathological appearance. When the criteria defined here are carefully applied, accurate diagnoses can be made in most circumstances. It is important to recognize this neoplasm and its simulators histologically so that proper treatment can be instituted.

SUMMARY

Kaposi's sarcoma is the neoplasm most commonly associated with HIV infection. Since its presence in the proper clinical context is an AIDS defining event, histopathological confirmation is often required for diagnosis. It is essential that clinicians know the criteria for histopathological diagnosis. When the criteria outlined are followed, the diagnosis can be made with certainty in most cases. A number of conditions may simulate KS both clinically and histologically, and it is important that those who care for patients with HIV infection are aware of these.

References

Ackerman AB (1979) Subtle clues to conventional microscopy: the patch stage of Kaposi's sarcoma. *American Journal of Dermatopathology* **1** 165–172

Amazon K and Rywlin AM (1979) Subtle clues to the diagnosis by conventional microscopy: lymph node involvement in Kaposi's sarcoma. *American Journal of Dermatopathology* **1** 173

Amazon K and Rywlin AM (1988) Systemic manifestations, In: Gottlieb GJ and Ackerman AB (eds). *Kaposi's Sarcoma: A Text and Atlas*, pp 113–129, Lea and Febiger, Philadelphia

Barbanti-Brodano G, Pagnani M, Viadana P, Beth-Giraldo E and Giraldo G (1987) BK virus DNA in Kaposi's sarcoma. *Antibiotics and Chemotherapy (Basel)* **38** 113–120

Berger TG, Tappero JW, Kaymen A and LeBoit PE (1989) Bacillary (epithelioid) angiomatosis and concurrent Kaposi's sarcoma in acquired immunodeficiency syndrome. *Archives of Dermatology* **125** 1543–1547

Centers for Disease Control (1985) Revision of the case definition of acquired immunodeficiency syndrome for national reporting United States. *Morbidity and Mortality Weekly Report* **34** 373–375

Chachoua A, Krigel RL, Lafleur F *et al* (1989) Prognostic factors and staging classification of patients with epidemic Kaposi's sarcoma. *Journal of Clinical Oncology* **7** 774–780

Cockerell CJ and Le Boit PE (1990) Bacillary angiomatosis: a newly characterized, pseudoneoplastic, infectious, cutaneous vascular disorder. *Journal of American Academy of Dermatology* **22** 501–512

Dictor M and Jarplid B (1988) The cause of Kaposi's sarcoma: an avian retroviral analog. *Journal of American Academy of Dermatology* **18** 398–402

Drew ML, Mills J, Hauer LB, Miner RC and Rutherford GW (1988) Declining prevalence of Kaposi's sarcoma in homosexual AIDS patients paralleled by fall in cytomegalovirus transmission. *Lancet* **i** 66

Friedman-Kien AE, Saltzman BR, Cao YZ *et al* (1990) Kaposi's sarcoma in HIV-negative homosexual men. *Lancet* **335** 168–169

Gottlieb GJ and Ackerman AB (1988) *Kaposi's Sarcoma: A Text and Atlas*, pp 29–113. Lea and Febiger, Philadelphia

Grody WW, Lewin KJ and Naeim F (1988) Detection of cytomegalovirus DNA in classic and epidemic Kaposi's sarcoma by in situ hybridization. *Human Pathology* **19** 524–526

Hennessey NP, Friedman-Kien AE (1989) Clinical simulators of the lesions of Kaposi's sarcoma, In: Friedman-Kien AE (ed). *Color Atlas of AIDS*, pp 49–71, WB Saunders, Philadelphia

Lever WF and Schaumburg-Lever G (1983) *Histopathology of the Skin* 6th ed, pp 636–640. JP Lippincott Co, Philadelphia

Longo DL, Steis RG, Lane HC *et al* (1984) Malignancies in the AIDS patient: Natural history, treatment strategies and preliminary results, In: Selikoff IJ, Teirstein AS and Hirschman SZ (eds). "Acquired Immune Deficiency Syndrome", *Annals of New York Academy of Sciences* **437** 421–429

Lubin J and Rywlin AM (1971) Lymphoma-like lymph node changes in Kaposi's sarcoma. *Archives of Pathology* **92** 338

McDougall JK, Olson KA, Smith PP and Collier AC (1987) Detection of cytomegalovirus and AIDS-associated retrovirus in tissues of patients with AIDS, Kaposi's sarcoma and persistent lymphadenopathy. *Antibiotics and Chemotherapy (Basel)* **38** 99–112

Muggia FM and Lonberg M (1986) Kaposi's sarcoma and AIDS. *Medical Clinics of North America* **70** 139–154

Niedt GW and Schinella RA (1985) Acquired immunodeficiency syndrome: clinicopathological study of 56 autopsies. *Archives of Pathology and Laboratory Medicine* **109** 727–734

Rappersberger K, Tschachler E, Zonzits E *et al* (1990) Endemic Kaposi's sarcoma in human immunodeficiency virus type 1 seronegative persons: demonstration of retrovirus-like particles in cutaneous lesions. *Journal of Investigative Dermatology* **95** 371–381

Ruszczak Z, da Silva AM and Orfanos CE (1987) Angioproliferative changes in clinically non-involved, perilesional skin in AIDS-associated Kaposi's sarcoma. *Dermatologicala* **175** 270–279

Safai B, Johnson KG, Myskowski PL *et al* (1985) The natural history of Kaposi's sarcoma in the acquired immunodeficiency syndrome. *Annals of Internal Medicine* **103** 744–750

Salahuddin SZ, Nakamura S, Biberfeld P *et al* (1988) Angiogenic properties of Kaposi's sarcoma-derived cells after long-term culture in vitro. *Science* **242** 430–433

Santucci M, Pimpinelli N, Moretti S and Giannotti B (1988) Classic and immunodeficiency-associated Kaposi's sarcoma. *Archives of Pathology and Laboratory Medicine* **112** 1214–1220

Taylor J, Afrasiabi R, Fahey JL *et al* (1986) Prognostically significant classification of immune changes in AIDS with Kaposi's sarcoma. *Blood* **67** 666–671

The author is responsible for the accuracy of the references.

Epidemiology of HIV Associated Non-Hodgkin Lymphoma

G I OBRAMS[1] • S GRUFFERMAN[2]

[1]*Epidemiology and Biostatistics Program, National Cancer Institute,*
Bethesda, Maryland 20892;
[2]*Department of Clinical Epidemiology and Preventive Medicine,*
University of Pittsburgh School of Medicine,
Pittsburgh, Pennsylvania 15213

INTRODUCTION

Non-Hodgkin lymphoma (NHL) is a group of neoplasms of the lymphoreticular system, but its classification has been a source of confusion and controversy over the years. The working formulation developed under a project sponsored by the National Cancer Institute is currently the most widely used classification system (Non-Hodgkin's Pathology Lymphoma Classification Project, 1982).

Non-Hodgkin lymphoma has been relatively uncommon in the USA, with age adjusted incidence rates of 5.8 per 100 000 per year for white males and a male to female ratio of 1.4:1 (Greene, 1982). Incidence rates in Western countries have shown an upward trend since 1960. The Surveillance, Epidemiology and End Results (SEER) program database of the National Cancer Institute registers the incident cases of cancer in areas comprising 10% of the US population. The SEER program has shown a steady increase in the incidence of +NHL: from 1973 to 1987, there was a 50% increase in the incidence of NHL

(Ries *et al*, 1990). From 1973 to 1984, there was a 2.7-fold increase in the incidence of primary brain lymphoma (Eby *et al*, 1988).

An association of NHL with HIV infection was recognized about a year later than that for Kaposi's sarcoma (KS). In 1982, an unusual outbreak of Burkitt's like lymphoma (BL like) was described among homosexual men in San Francisco (Ziegler *et al*, 1982); similar observations were made in Los Angeles (Levine *et al*, 1984). The first extended series of NHL in homosexual men was reported in 1984 (Ziegler *et al*, 1984). The excess of high grade NHL among "never-married men" was first documented in 1985 (Biggar *et al*, 1985). The category "never-married men" was used to approximate the category "homosexual men". That 21% of the lymphomas in these young homosexual men were preceded by KS, that the majority of AIDS cases in the USA were in young homosexual men and that NHL was rare among the young before this epidemic suggested that these NHL cases were AIDS related. A series of 18 NHL cases in homosexual men was reported from New York City (Ioachim *et al*, 1985), and the lymphomas were noted to be high grade and B cell. Subsequent studies from New York confirmed these clinical findings among HIV infected individuals with NHL (Ahmed *et al*, 1987; Kaplan *et al*, 1987). Non-Hodgkin lymphoma occurred as a second malignancy in AIDS patients who originally presented with KS (and vice versa), and a second, clonally discrete NHL has occurred in individuals who originally presented with B cell lymphoma (Barriga *et al*, 1988).

The observation of excess NHL among individuals with AIDS is consistent with the increased risk of lymphoma in other immunodeficiency states. Therapeutically immunosuppressed patients such as recipients of organ transplants have a 30- to 300-fold increased risk of lymphomas (Hoover and Fraumeni, 1973; Penn, 1986, 1988, 1990). Acquired autoimmune disorders such as Sjögren's syndrome and congenital immunodeficiency states such as Wiscott-Aldrich syndrome are also associated with an excess incidence of malignant lymphomas (Freter, 1990). Therefore, it is not surprising to encounter an increased risk for lymphomas among individuals with HIV infection. It remains to be determined what specific alterations in immune function confer an increased risk of NHL. The immunological abnormalities in patients with HIV associated lymphoma have been reported to be similar to those in AIDS patients presenting with KS or opportunistic infections (Gill *et al*, 1985), although specific functional immunological abnormalities remain to be investigated.

CASE DEFINITION

HIV infected individuals have a clinical presentation of NHL similar to that seen in therapeutically immunosuppressed patients, in primary immunodeficiency states and in allograft recipients (Brusamolino *et al*, 1989). Rapid progression and short survival are common.

In a series of 90 homosexual men with lymphoma (Ziegler *et al*, 1984) 62%

had high grade subtypes, and immunoblastic sarcoma and Burkitt's lymphoma accounted for 60% of all histological types. Most of these men presented with tumours in extranodal sites, including bone marrow, central nervous system (CNS) and intra-abdominal involvement. In a series of 29 homosexual men with malignant lymphoma in the Los Angeles area, systemic symptoms consisting of fever, weight loss and night sweats were common at diagnosis (76%) (Levine et al, 1985). Half of the patients complained of significant fatigue. Extranodal disease was present in 86% of the patients, as compared with a prior series of non-AIDS NHL patients in which only 1% had extranodal disease. Initial CNS involvement was detected in 28% of these patients. These findings are more striking in view of the fact that some of the cases in these series were quite likely unrelated to AIDS. Two other large series of lymphoid neoplasms associated with AIDS were described at New York University (Knowles et al, 1988) and in Italy (Italian Cooperative Group for AIDS-related Tumors, 1988), and the findings were similar to those reported from the earlier series.

In summary, more than half of these patients presented with lymphomas of high grade histology, evenly distributed between small non-cleaved (including Burkitt's) and large cell immunoblastic lymphomas.

Another distinguishing clinical feature of HIV associated lymphomas was occurrence in extranodal sites. Presenting sites included the rectum (Burkes et al, 1986), liver (Lisker-Melman et al, 1989), heart (Gill et al, 1987), bone marrow (Levine et al 1985), oral mucosa (Green and Eversole, 1989; Hintner et al, 1989; Kaugars and Burns, 1989; Raphael et al, 1990) and gastrointestinal tract (Gianfelice et al, 1987). Primary CNS lymphoma may account for a quarter of all HIV associated NHL, and involvement of the CNS occurs in 10–25% of patients presenting with other primary sites. Recognition of CNS lymphoma is difficult, since CNS toxoplasmosis and progressive multifocal leukoencephalopathy may have similar presentations (Snider et al, 1983).

Because of these clinical observations, the case definition initially chosen as diagnostic of AIDS was modified to include HIV positive patients with high grade B cell lymphoma and primary brain lymphomas (Centers for Disease Control, 1985).

Lymphoma may often be occult in AIDS, as demonstrated by a necropsy series of 20 patients with HIV associated lymphoma. In 3 of the 8 patients with primary CNS lymphoma, the diagnosis was established only at necropsy; 3 of 12 systemic lymphomas were diagnosed only at necropsy (Loureiro et al, 1988). Eleven percent of AIDS patients who underwent necropsy at the University of Southern California between 1982 and 1987 were found to have previously undiagnosed lymphomas (Klatt, 1988). In a series of necropsies of AIDS patients in New York City between 1981 and 1987, 8 of 20 (40%) lymphomas diagnosed at necropsy were not suspected before death (Wilkes et al, 1988). These series may have been biased by the reason for necropsy, and some of the missed diagnoses occurred early in the AIDS epidemic, but the concern remains that the incidence of HIV associated NHL may well be higher than that ascertained on the basis of clinical diagnosis.

DESCRIPTIVE EPIDEMIOLOGY

Incidence Statistics

Estimates of the incidence of HIV associated NHL have been difficult to develop without knowing the size of the groups at risk. The analysis of HIV associated increases in NHL incidence is also complicated by the increases in the incidence of NHL that are occurring independently of HIV infection.

Various sources of data have been analyzed to ascertain the effect of the HIV epidemic on the incidence of NHL in the USA. Most investigators have reported a 5% to 10% incidence of NHL among persons infected with HIV, in about 3% as a primary AIDS diagnosis. In 1985, an analysis of the data collected by the SEER program in San Francisco demonstrated a significant increase in the morbidity odds ratio (MOR 9:1) for high grade lymphomas among "never-married men" in this metropolitan area comparing the period 1973–1980 with 1981–1982 (Biggar et al, 1985). In the same year, data from the University of Southern California Cancer Surveillance Program, the population based cancer registry for Los Angeles County, indicated a 60% increase since 1981 in the incidence of B cell immunoblastic sarcoma and small cell non-cleaved lymphoma (either BL or BL like) in never-married men (Ross et al, 1985). Similar findings were reported in 1988 in another study from the San Francisco area (Harnly et al, 1988), noting a fivefold increase between 1980 and 1985 in the incidence of NHL among never-married men living in census tracts with a high rate of AIDS. This increase continued through 1986 (Horn et al, 1989). In the USA, New York City has had the largest number of individuals at risk for AIDS for the longest period of time. In a study from the New York State Cancer Registry, the incidence of NHL increased in New York City between 1980 and 1984, most notably in neighbourhoods with a high AIDS incidence (Kristal et al, 1988). A comparison of NHL incidence rates in 1973–1976 with 1985 for never-married men in New York City showed a sixfold increase in that period. The most striking increases occurred for Burkitt's lymphoma and immunoblastic lymphoma incidence rates (Biggar et al, 1989). An analysis of SEER data demonstrated a tenfold increase in the incidence of NHL among never-married men aged 20–49 from 1973–1978 to 1985–1987 in the San Francisco area. The increase in high grade NHL in this group was over 100-fold (Rabkin and Goedert, 1990).

These trends indicate that the incidence of NHL has increased in parallel with the evolution of the AIDS epidemic. Only a few analyses, however, have focused on persons at risk for HIV infection and AIDS other than "never-married" (meaning homosexual) men. In a study of New York State prisoners who were intravenous drug abusers, a 40-fold higher incidence of NHL than in the general population was reported (Ahmed et al, 1987). Among 1753 HIV positive haemophiliacs at 20 USA haemophilia treatment centres, AIDS has developed in 301. Of these AIDS patients, 18 (6%) had lymphoma by 1989 (Ragni et al, 1989). Histologically, these were high or intermediate grade tumours, and 77% presented at extranodal sites.

It is of interest to ascertain what proportion of NHL cases are now associated with HIV infection. In a study of the incident cases of NHL reported to the Atlanta SEER program in 1989, sera were tested for HIV infection; 41% of high grade NHL were HIV seropositive, compared with 6% of other lymphomas, giving an indication of the importance of HIV infection as a risk factor for NHL and confirming the association of high grade lymphomas with HIV (Liff *et al*, 1990).

Patient Characteristics

Lymphoma occurs among all groups of patients at risk of AIDS, including homosexual men, infants and children of HIV infected mothers (Andiman *et al*, 1985), intravenous drug users (Barbieri *et al*, 1986), patients with thalassaemia who receive multiple transfusions (Di Carlo *et al*, 1986) and spouses of HIV infected transfusion recipients (Duncan *et al*, 1986). No difference was seen between intravenous drug users and homosexual men with regard to NHL pathological type, grade or disease progression in the Italian Cooperative Group Study on AIDS-related Tumors (Vaccher *et al*, 1990).

Most people with AIDS related lymphoma are much younger than those with NHL not related to HIV infection (Levine, 1987). The median age in one case series was 37 years, with an age distribution identical to that for cases of AIDS reported to the Centers for Disease Control (CDC) (Ziegler *et al*, 1984).

The CDC have developed a national AIDS case report form for the USA with data collected by state and local health departments. The total number of lymphoma cases reported to the CDC by June, 1989, was 2824, which was 3% of all AIDS cases (Beral *et al*, 1991). A similar percentage has been reported from Europe (Casabona *et al*, 1991). One-fifth of the USA NHL cases were primary CNS lymphomas, and another fifth were Burkitt's lymphomas. The overall risk of NHL with AIDS was about 60 times that in the general population. The occurrence of NHL with AIDS varied by type of lymphoma, age, sex, race and risk group (Beral *et al*, 1991). AIDS associated immunoblastic lymphoma increased steadily with age; primary CNS lymphoma was constant at all ages; and Burkitt's lymphoma peaked at ages 10–19. Non-Hodgkin lymphoma was more common in men with AIDS (3.1%) than in women (1.4%) and in whites (3.7%) than in blacks (1.4%). Adjusting for age, sex and race, NHL was more common in haemophiliacs (5.2%) than in homosexuals (3.4%) and least common in individuals born in Africa or the Caribbean (1.0%).

In a project linking the Illinois AIDS registry (1983–1987) with the Cancer registry (1985–1987), 87 of 2528 AIDS cases (3.4%) had NHL. The individuals with NHL were similar to other persons with AIDS with regard to age, sex, place of residence and AIDS risk factors. The proportion of AIDS cases with NHL did not change over time. The standardized incidence ratio for NHL in persons with AIDS (compared with NHL in the general population of Illinois and with men in SEER states) was 140, which was a statistically significant increase in risk (Cote *et al*, 1991).

Geographical Patterns

In the USA, no systematic variation by state of residence or by country of birth was found in the frequency of NHL among individuals with AIDS reported to the CDC (Beral *et al*, 1991).

Among other countries that have reported data on the frequency of NHL among AIDS patients, there are no striking differences. In Denmark, of 358 AIDS patients registered by 1988, 7.5% had lymphoma (Hamilton-Dutoit *et al*, 1989). In Mexico, in a necropsy series of 177 consecutive patients with AIDS, 9% had NHL (Mohar *et al*, 1990). Of 22 Italian patients (largely intravenous drug users) with AIDS whose brains were examined at necropsy, 3 were found to have primary CNS lymphoma (Gianpalmo *et al*, 1989).

Patterns Over Time

The status of HIV associated NHL patients has been changing over time. In the series reported in 1984, 47% of the patients with NHL had a previous diagnosis of KS, opportunistic infection or both, and only 15% had no previous AIDS diagnosis (Ziegler *et al*, 1984). In a more recent series in San Francisco, 37% of patients had no preceding AIDS related diagnosis (Kaplan *et al*, 1989). In one Washington area study of patients treated in the past 2 years, 58% had no previous AIDS diagnosis (Freter, 1990). These changes may be due to earlier recognition of HIV infection, changes in risk factors or an impact of anti-retroviral or anti-pneumocystis therapy.

The role of anti-retroviral therapies in NHL incidence is under investigation. In one series, a high grade B cell lymphoma developed in 8 of 55 HIV infected patients on long term azidothymidine (AZT) regimens (Pluda *et al*, 1990. The estimated probability of developing lymphoma by the 36th month of therapy was 46%, and the risk of NHL was approximately 10% per year of advanced HIV infection. Prolonged survival in the setting of immunosuppression with T4 depletion (to fewer than 50 T4 cells/ mm^3) was thought to be an important factor in the development of these lymphomas. Although a direct role of AZT cannot be ruled out, this is unlikely, since these lymphomas were of the same type as those that develop in association with untreated HIV infection.

In a cohort of homosexual men from New York and Washington, the NHL incidence per year increased from 0.8% in 1984 to 2.6% in 1988. The cumulative incidence rate in 10 years was 18% (Rabkin and Goedert, 1990). In preliminary data from the Multicenter AIDS Cohort Study, which includes homosexual men in four USA areas, the lymphomas have shown a significant upward trend in incidence between 1985 and 1989 (Vermund S, personal communication).

The impact of HIV infection on the numbers of NHL cases each year has been estimated through modeling approaches. In 1990, about 2000 HIV associated NHL cases occurred in the USA (Rabkin *et al*, 1991). Projections of AIDS case numbers in the USA, developed with the back calculation method

(Gail and Brookmeyer, 1988), suggest that from 2900 to 9800 HIV associated lymphomas may occur in the USA in 1992 (Gail *et al*, 1991) and that this will represent between 8% and 27% of the 36 000 NHL cases diagnosed in the USA in 1992.

EPIDEMIOLOGICAL STUDIES

Beyond the acceptance of HIV associated NHL as an AIDS defining condition and the demonstration of an increasing incidence of NHL, nearly all research directed towards the identification of specific risk factors or viral cofactors in NHL development is still in an early phase.

A better understanding of the epidemiology of non-HIV associated lymphomas, especially high grade subtypes, is needed to develop further research on HIV associated cases. Case control studies of NHL not associated with HIV infection have reported increased risks among individuals with histories of steroid use, hives or eczema (Cartwright *et al*, 1988), rural residence (Barnes *et al*, 1987), occupational exposures, including agricultural pesticides and herbicides (Pearce *et al*, 1985, 1986, 1987; Hoar *et al*, 1986) and relatively high radiation exposures (Beebe *et al*, 1978). As noted earlier, there is a well established relationship between various states of immune abnormality, receipt of immunosuppressive drugs and an increased risk for NHL, although the specific functional immunological abnormalities associated with this increase in risk remain to be defined. Burkitt's lymphoma, primarily the endemic form, has been associated with prior Epstein-Barr virus (EBV) infection and with the presence of EBV nuclear antigen and DNA within tumour cells (Ziegler *et al*, 1976; de Thé *et al*, 1978).

Ongoing epidemiological research projects include a population based case control study of NHL in the San Francisco Bay area and another in the Los Angeles area, the latter focusing on HIV associated high grade lymphomas. In addition, cohorts of HIV infected individuals, including haemophiliacs and homosexual men, are being closely studied for HIV infection and its sequelae, including studies of the risk factors and incidence patterns of NHL development.

DISCUSSION

It is clear that an important new factor in the aetiology of NHL, namely, HIV infection, has emerged in recent years. Available data do not allow us to identify the precise aetiological mechanism, for example, whether it is the HIV virus per se or whether it is an aspect of the immunosuppression resulting from HIV infection. Nevertheless, it appears likely that the incidence of lymphomas will continue to rise in the HIV infected population, particularly as the clinical management of HIV disease improves, thereby extending the lifetime of HIV infected patients despite depression of immune function. Thus some of the gains in survival from AIDS may be offset by an increased risk for lymphomas.

Many important research questions remain to be answered. Foremost on the list of questions is an attempt to identify risk factors for the occurrence of NHL in HIV infected patients. Why do lymphomas develop in some patients with HIV infection or AIDS but not in others? Why do lymphomas develop in the CNS in some patients but at other anatomical sites in others? Are there genetic factors, clues in the family history of cancer or hormonal factors that modify the risk of NHL development? Intriguing leads are available from data that show higher risks for NHL for men than for women, for whites than for blacks and for haemophiliacs than for homosexual men. The second important quest is to characterize further the HIV associated lymphomas. Why do the HIV associated immunoblastic lymphomas increase in incidence with age, whereas the primary CNS lymphomas occur at equal frequency at all ages? Are these lymphomas polyclonal or monoclonal? Is there evidence of involvement of oncogenes such as c-*myc* or tumour suppressor genes such as p53? Such data will provide important aetiological leads. The third question is how to define the relationship between EBV and NHL. It is becoming evident that many of the primary CNS lymphomas are EBV associated. In EBV associated tumours, is the virus in a latent or replicative phase? How do risk factors differ between EBV associated and non-EBV associated tumours? Are other viral cofactors involved, for example, human herpesvirus type 6? Why does HIV associated NHL, like lymphomas seen in other immunosuppressed states, have a predilection for extranodal sites? Related to this may be the observation that NHL, particularly of the CNS, is increasing in the general population. Another interesting question relates to the observation of lymphoma of the eye in association with occult CNS lymphoma and which functional aspects of immune function affect risk for lymphoma in anatomical sites that are "immunologically privileged", with a paucity of cells of the immune system (Schanzer *et al*, 1991). Finally, what is the effect on the incidence of HIV associated NHL (and its clinical manifestations and progression) of the increasingly widespread use of AZT?

Many of the questions posed above can be answered by careful epidemiological case control studies. Certain special populations such as the Multicenter AIDS Cohort Study that is supported by the National Institute of Allergy and Infectious Diseases and the National Cancer Institute particularly lend themselves to the conduct of nested case control studies. Subjects in such populations have been followed closely and sequentially over time, with the collection and storage of biological specimens. Subjects in whom lymphoma has developed can be identified and matched with comparable HIV infected or HIV negative controls from the same cohort to see how the cases and controls differ. As lymphomas develop, information will be gained that may help us intervene in earlier stages of NHL development both in HIV infected individuals and perhaps in individuals not infected with HIV.

Will the answers to these questions lend themselves to preventive strategies? Our guess is that the most important preventive measure that can be taken is the prevention of initial HIV infection. As the available therapeutic armamentarium grows, it may be possible to intervene on specific immunological abnormalities that are risk factors for lymphomas.

In conclusion, we are in the midst of an alarming and scientifically fascinating epidemic of NHL related to the worldwide epidemic of AIDS. Comprehensive research efforts to learn more about the contributing factors and causes of HIV associated lymphomas are likely to shed important new light on the epidemiology and aetiology of lymphoreticular malignancies in general and perhaps a variety of other cancers as well.

SUMMARY

The excess of NHL associated with HIV infection is well established. Clinically, HIV associated NHL is characterized by histological evidence of a high grade of malignancy, B cell origin, extensive extranodal involvement (most notably of the CNS) and poor prognosis. High grade B cell lymphoma or primary brain lymphoma in HIV infected individuals is considered diagnostic of AIDS by the Centers for Disease Control. The incidence of NHL among individuals with AIDS varies by subtype of lymphoma, age, sex, race and risk group. Younger individuals, males, whites and haemophiliacs are at higher risk than other groups. The incidence of HIV associated NHL is increasing. Because of the paucity of data on risk factors for this malignancy, the current possibilities for risk modification are limited to the prevention of HIV infection.

Acknowledgements

We thank Dr Robert Biggar, Dr Joseph F. Fraumeni Jr, Dr Elizabeth Holly and Dr Daniela Seminara for their thoughtful comments and suggestions.

References

Ahmed T, Wormser GP, Stahl RE et al (1987) Malignant lymphomas in a population at risk for acquired immune deficiency syndrome. *Cancer* **60** 719–723

Andiman WA, Eastman R, Martin K et al (1985) Opportunistic lymphoproliferations associated with Epstein-Barr viral DNA in infants and children with AIDS. *Lancet* **ii** 1390–1393

Barbieri D, Gualandi M, Tassinari MC, Scapoli G and Guerra G (1986) B-cell lymphomas in two seropositive heroin addicts. *Lancet* **ii** 1039

Barriga F, Whang-Peng J, Lee E et al (1988) Development of a second clonally discrete Burkitt's lymphoma in a human immunodeficiency virus-positive homosexual patient. *Blood* **72** 792–795

Barnes N, Cartwright RA, O'Brien C, Roberts B, Richards IDG and Hopkinson JM (1987) Variation in lymphoma incidence within Yorkshire health region. *British Journal of Cancer* **55** 81–84

Beebe GW, Kato H and Land C (1978) Studies of the mortality of A-bomb survivors 6. Mortality and radiation dose, 1950–1974. *Radiation Research* **75** 138–201

Beral V, Peterman T, Berkelman R and Jaffe H (1991) Epidemiology of AIDS associated non-Hodgkin's lymphoma. *Lancet* **337** 805–809

Biggar RJ, Horm J, Lubin JH, Goedert JJ, Greene MH and Fraumeni JF Jr (1985) Cancer trends in a population at risk of acquired immunodeficiency syndrome. *Journal of the National Cancer Institute* **74** 793–797

Biggar RJ, Burnett W, Mikl J and Nasca P (1989) Cancer among New York men at risk of acquired immunodeficiency syndrome. *International Journal of Cancer* **43** 979–985

Brusamolino E, Pagnucco G and Bernasconi C (1989) Secondary lymphomas—a review on lymphoproliferative diseases arising in immunocompromised hosts: prevalence, clinical features and pathogenetic mechanisms. *Haematologica* **74** 605–622

Burkes RL, Meyer PR, Gill PS, Parker JW, Rasheed S and Levine AM (1986) Rectal lymphoma in homosexual men. *Archives of Internal Medicine* **146** 913–915

Cartwright RA, McKinney PA, O'Brien C *et al* (1988) Non-Hodgkin's lymphoma: case-control epidemiological study in Yorkshire. *Leukemia Research* **12** 81–88

Casabona J, Melbye M, Biggar RJ and the AIDS Registry Contributors (1991) Kaposi's sarcoma and non-Hodgkin's lymphoma in European AIDS cases. *International Journal of Cancer* **47** 49–53

Centers for Disease Control (1985) Case definition of AIDS revised. *Morbidity and Mortality Weekly Reports* **43** 373–375

Cote TR, Howe HL, Anderson SP, Martin RJ, Evans E and Francis BJ (1991) A systematic consideration of the neoplastic spectrum of AIDS: registry linkage in Illinois. *AIDS* **5** 49–53

de Thé G, Geser A, Day NE *et al* (1978) Epidemiological evidence for causal relationship between Epstein-Barr virus and Burkitt's lymphoma: results of the Ugandan prospective study. *Nature* **274** 756–761

Di Carlo EF, Amberson JB, Metroka CE, Ballard P, Moore A and Mouradian JA (1986) Malignant lymphomas and the acquired immunodeficiency syndrome. *Archives of Pathology and Laboratory Medicine* **11** 1012–1016

Duncan ED, Miller HJ and McKeever WP (1986) Non-Hodgkin's lymphoma, HTLV-III/LAV, and HTLV-III/LAV antibody in the wife of a man with transfusion-acquired AIDS. *American Journal of Medicine* **81** 898–900

Eby NL, Grufferman S, Flannely CM, Schold SC, Vogel S and Burger PC (1988) Increasing incidence of primary brain lymphoma in the US. *Cancer* **62** 2461–2465

Freter C (1990) Acquired immunodeficiency syndrome-associated lymphomas. *National Cancer Institute Monographs* **10** 45–54

Gail MH and Brookmeyer R (1988) Methods for projecting course of acquired immunodeficiency syndrome epidemic. *Journal of the National Cancer Institute* **80** 900–911

Gail MH, Pluda JM, Rabkin CS *et al* (1991) Projections of the incidence of AIDS-related non-Hodgkin's lymphoma. *Journal of the National Cancer Institute* **83** 695–701

Gianfelice D, Tosenthall L and Falutz J (1987) Gallium-67 detection of occult gastric lymphoma in AIDS. *American Journal of Radiology* **149** 305–306

Gianpalmo A, Pesce C, Ardoino S, Provaggi MA and Quaglia AC (1989) Neuropathological findings in an autopsy series of Italian subjects with AIDS. *Clinical Neuropathology* **8** 120–125

Gill PS, Levine AM, Meyer PR *et al* (1985) Primary central nervous system lymphoma in homosexual men. *American Journal of Medicine* **78** 742–748

Gill PS, Chandraratna AN, Meyer P and Levine AM (1987) Malignant lymphoma: cardiac involvement at initial presentation. *Journal of Clinical Oncology* **5** 216–224

Green TL and Eversole LR (1989) Oral lymphomas in HIV-infected patients: association with Epstein-Barr virus DNA. *Oral Surgery, Oral Medicine, and Oral Pathology* **67** 437–442

Greene MH (1982) Non-Hodgkin's lymphoma and mycosis fungoides, In: Schottenfeld D and Fraumeni JF Jr (eds). *Cancer Epidemiology and Prevention*, pp 754–778, WB Saunders Company, Philadelphia, Pennsylvania

Hamilton-Dutoit SJ, Pallesen G, Karkov J, Skinhoj P, Franzmann M and Pedersen C (1989) Identification of EBV-DNA in tumour cells of AIDS-related lymphomas by in-situ hybridization. *Lancet* **ii** 554–555

Harnly ME, Swan SH, Holly EA, Kelter A and Padian N (1988) Temporal trends in the incidence of non-Hodgkin's lymphoma and selected malignancies in a population with a high incidence of acquired immunodeficiency syndrome (AIDS). *American Journal of Epidemiology* **128** 261–267

Hintner H and Fritsch P (1989) Skin neoplasia in the immunodeficient host. *Current Problems in Dermatology* **18** 210–217

Hoar SK, Blair A, Holmes FF, Boysen CD, Robel RJ, Hoover R and Fraumeni JF Jr (1986) Agricultural herbicide use and risk of lymphoma and soft-tissue sarcoma. *Journal of the American Medical Association* **256** 1141–1147

Hoover R and Fraumeni JF Jr (1973) Risk of cancer in renal transplant recipients. *Lancet* **ii** 55–57

Horn PL, DeLorenza GN, Brown SR, Holly EA and West DW (1989) Re: "Temporal trends in the incidence of non-Hodgkin's lymphoma and selected malignancies in a population with a high incidence of acquired immunodeficiency syndrome" (letter). *American Journal of Epidemiology* **130** 1069–1071

Ioachim HL, Cooper MC and Hellman GC (1985) Lymphomas in men at high risk for acquired immunodeficiency syndrome (AIDS): a study of 18 cases. *Cancer* **56** 2831–2842

Italian Cooperative Group for AIDS-related Tumors (1988) Malignant lymphomas in patients with or at risk for AIDS in Italy. *Journal of the National Cancer Institute* **80** 855–860

Kaplan MH, Susin M, Pahwa SG *et al* (1987) Neoplastic complications of HTLV-III infection: lymphomas and solid tumors. *American Journal of Medicine* **82** 389–396

Kaplan LD, Abrams DI, Feigal E *et al* (1989) AIDS-associated non-Hodgkin's lymphoma in San Francisco. *Journal of the American Medical Association* **261** 719–724

Kaugars GE and Burns JC (1989) Non-Hodgkin's lymphoma of the oral cavity associated with AIDS. *Oral Surgery, Oral Medicine, and Oral Pathology* **67** 433–436

Klatt EC (1988) Diagnostic findings in patients with acquired immune deficiency syndrome (AIDS). *Journal of Acquired Immune Deficiency Syndromes* **1** 459–465

Knowles DM, Chamulak GA, Subar M *et al* (1988) Lymphoid neoplasia associated with the acquired immunodeficiency syndrome (AIDS): the New York University experience with 105 patients (1981–1986). *Annals of Internal Medicine* **108** 744–753

Kristal AR, Nasca PC, Burnett WS and Mikl J (1988) Changes in the epidemiology of non-Hodgkin's lymphoma associated with epidemic human immunodeficiency virus (HIV) infection. *American Journal of Epidemiology* **128** 711–718

Levine AM (1987) Non-Hodgkin's lymphomas and other malignancies in the acquired immunodeficiency syndrome. *Seminars in Oncology* **14 (Supplement)** 34–39

Levine AM, Meyer PR, Begandy MK *et al* (1984) Development of B-cell lymphoma in homosexual men: clinical and immunologic findings. *Annals of Internal Medicine* **100** 7–13

Levine AM, Gill PG and Rasheed S (1985) Human retrovirus-associated lymphoproliferative disorders in homosexual men. *Progress in Allergy* **37** 244–258

Levine AM, Burkes RL, Walker M *et al* (1985) B-cell lymphoma in two monogamous homosexual men. *Archives of Internal Medicine* **145** 479–481

Liff J, Eley JW, Khabbaz RF, Selik RM and Chan WC (1990) HIV-seropositivity and Hodgkin's lymphoma. *Fifth International Conference on AIDS*, San Francisco, California [Abstract]

Lisker-Melman M, Pittaluga S, Pluda JM *et al* (1989) Primary lymphoma of the liver in a patient with acquired immune deficiency syndrome and chronic hepatitis B. *American Journal of Gastroenterology* **84** 1445–1448

Loureiro C, Gill PS, Meyer PR, Rhodes R, Rarick MU and Levine AM (1988) Autopsy findings in AIDS-related lymphoma. *Cancer* **62** 735–739

Mohar A, Romo J, Salido F *et al* (1990) The clinical and autopsy spectrum of HIV infection in a consecutive series of autopsy patients seen in Mexico City. *Fifth International Conference on AIDS*, San Francisco, California [Abstract]

Non-Hodgkin's Lymphoma Pathology Classification Project (1982) National Cancer Institute sponsored study of classifications of non-Hodgkin's lymphomas. *Cancer* **49** 2112–2135

Pearce NE, Smith AH and Fischer DO (1985) Malignant lymphoma and multiple myeloma linked with agricultural occupations in a New Zealand Cancer Registry-based study. *American Journal of Epidemiology* **121** 225–237

Pearce NE, Smith AH, Howard JK, Sheppard RA, Giles HJ and Teague CA (1986) Non-Hodgkin's lymphoma and exposure to phenoxyherbicides, chlorophenols, fencing work and meat works employment: a case-control study. *British Journal of Industrial Medicine* **43** 75–83

Pearce NE, Sheppard RA, Smith AH and Teague CA (1987) Non-Hodgkin's lymphoma and farming: an expanded case-control study. *International Journal of Cancer* **39** 155–161

Pluda, JM, Yarchoan R, Jaffe ES *et al* (1990) Development of non-Hodgkin lymphoma in a cohort of patients with severe human immunodeficiency virus (HIV) infection on long-term antiretroviral therapy. *Annals of Internal Medicine* **113** 276–282

Penn I (1986) The occurrence of malignant tumors in immunosuppressed states. *Progress in Allergy* **37** 259–300

Penn I (1988) Tumors of the immunocompromised patient. *Annual Review of Medicine* **39** 63–73

Penn I (1990) Cancers complicating organ transplantation (editorial). *New England Journal of Medicine* **323** 1767–1769

Rabkin CS and Goedert JJ (1990) Risk of non-Hodgkin lymphoma and Kaposi's sarcoma in homosexual men (letter). *Lancet* **336** 248–249

Rabkin CS, Biggar RJ and Horm J (1991) Increasing incidence of cancers associated with the human immunodeficiency virus epidemic. *International Journal of Cancer* **47** 692–696

Ragni MV, Kingsley LA, Duzyk A, Obrams I and the HMS Study Group (1989) HIV-associated malignancy in hemophiliacs: preliminary report from the hemophilia malignancy study. *Blood* **74** 89a [Abstract]

Raphael M, Pallesen G, Chomette G, Audoin J, Szpirglas B, Hamilton-Dutoit S and Lenoir G (1990) Oral mucosal lymphomas in AIDS patients. *Fifth International Conference on AIDS*, San Francisco, California [Abstract]

Ries LA, Barrett MJ and Labbe RR (eds) (1990) *Cancer Statistics Review: 1973–1987*, p II.4. National Cancer Institute, Bethesda, Maryland

Ross R, Dworsky R, Paganini-Hill A, Levine A and Mack T (1985) Non-Hodgkin's lymphomas in never-married men in Los Angeles. *British Journal of Cancer* **52** 785–787

Schanzer MC, Font RL and O'Malley RE (1991) A primary ocular malignant lymphoproliferation associated with the acquired immune deficiency syndrome. *Ophthalmology* **98** 88–91

Snider WD, Simpson DM, Aronyk KE and Nielsen SL (1983) Primary lymphoma of the central nervous system associated with acquired immunodeficiency syndrome (letter). *New England Journal of Medicine* **203** 45

Vaccher E, Tirelli U, Errante D, Rizzardi G, Palmieri G and Monfardini S for the Italian Cooperative Group Study on AIDS-related Tumors (1990) HIV-related non-Hodgkin's lymphomas in Italy: intravenous drug users versus homosexual men. *Fifth International Conference on AIDS*, San Francisco, California (Abstract)

Wilkes MS, Fortin AH, Felix JC, Godwin TA and Thompson WG (1988) Value of necropsy in acquired immunodeficiency syndrome. *Lancet* **ii** 85–88

Ziegler JL, Anderson M, Klein G and Henle W (1976) Detection of Epstein-Barr virus DNA in American Burkitt's lymphoma. *International Journal of Cancer* **17** 701–706

Ziegler JL, Drew WL, Miner RC *et al* (1982) Outbreak of Burkitt's-like lymphoma in homosexual men. *Lancet* **ii** 631–633

Ziegler JL, Beckstead JA, Volberding PA *et al* (1984) Non-Hodgkin's lymphoma in 90 homosexual men: relationship to generalized lymphadenopathy and acquired immunodeficiency syndrome. *New England Journal of Medicine* **311** 565–570

The authors are responsible for the accuracy of the references.

Aetiology and Pathogenesis of Non-Hodgkin Lymphoma in AIDS

J C LUXTON[1] • J A THOMAS[2] • D H CRAWFORD[1]

[1]*London School of Hygiene and Tropical Medicine, Keppel St., London;* [2]*Imperial Cancer Research Fund, Lincoln's Inn Fields, London*

INTRODUCTION

Since the early 1980s, following the first report of Burkitt's like lymphoma (BL like) in homosexual men (Ziegler *et al*, 1982), there has been a steady increase in the reported incidence of non-Hodgkin lymphoma (NHL) developing in patients with AIDS. Recognition of this clinical association with HIV infection (Ziegler *et al*, 1984) has led to the inclusion of NHL as one of the diagnostic criteria for AIDS (Centers for Disease Control, 1985). In a recent epidemiological survey, the frequency of NHL developing in association with AIDS has been estimated to be about 60 times greater than histologically similar lymphomas arising spontaneously in the general population. The incidence appears to vary with age and within specific risk groups for HIV infection (Beral *et al*, 1991). AIDS related NHLs (AIDS-NHL) are primarily of B cell origin, manifesting a variety of histological appearances. A summary of four major histopathological studies (Ziegler *et al*, 1984; Knowles *et al*, 1988; Levine *et al*, 1988; Lowenthal *et al*, 1988) by Levine (1990) shows that the majority of these tumours have high grade histological patterns consistent with diffuse immunoblastic large cell lymphoma, whereas significant but smaller numbers of these tumours have the appearance of small non-cleaved lymphoma or classical BL. Fewer patients develop intermediate, and even fewer low grade, types of NHL.

AIDS related NHLs show clinicohistological similarities to both BL, which has a well established association with Epstein-Barr virus (EBV), and a recently recognized group of EBV induced lymphoproliferative conditions arising in iatrogenically immunosuppressed individuals following organ and bone marrow transplantation. The demonstration of EBV DNA and EBV gene expression in a proportion of AIDS-NHLs by Southern blotting, cytohybridization and immunocytochemical techniques (Subar *et al*, 1988; Haluska *et al*, 1989) suggests that the involvement of EBV may be a necessary factor in the pathogenesis of disease in this particular group of NHL patients in whom altered or suppressed immune function is a common underlying factor. The severe immunosuppression that accompanies HIV infection renders infected individuals vulnerable to ubiquitous infectious agents. The capacity for EBV to produce polyclonal B cell activation and immortalize normal B cells into permanent B lymphoblastoid cell lines (BLCL) in vitro is therefore relevant to the pathogenesis of lymphoproliferative tumours arising in an immunosuppressed setting. The failure of EBV specific immunological responses in vivo may allow uncontrolled proliferation of EBV infected B cells. However, since these tumours do not develop in all AIDS patients, are not universally associated with EBV and may not be accompanied by overt immune deficiency, other factors have been implicated in the development of AIDS related NHL.

This chapter will therefore give an overview of the types of NHL seen in AIDS with particular reference to current concepts of their pathogenesis.

EPSTEIN-BARR VIRUS AND IMMUNE CONTROL

Epstein-Barr virus is a human herpesvirus that infects B lymphocytes (Pattengale *et al*, 1973) and squamous epithelial cells (Sixbey *et al*, 1984) and is associated with diseases of both cell types. It is the causative agent of infectious mononucleosis (Henle *et al*, 1968), a benign, self-limiting B lymphoproliferative disease, and is associated with B cell tumours such as BL (Lenoir, 1986), post-transplant lymphomas (Crawford *et al*, 1981) and nasopharyngeal carcinoma of epithelial origin (Epstein, 1978). This chapter will review the B cell tumours that are aetiologically linked to EBV.

Epstein-Barr Virus Infection In Vitro

Infection by EBV is initiated by the binding of the viral envelope glycoprotein gp340 to the CD21 molecule, the receptor for the C3d component of complement CR2 (Fingeroth *et al*, 1984), which is present on all mature B lymphocytes and a subpopulation of squamous epithelial cells (Sixbey *et al*,

1987). Infected epithelial cells undergo a lytic infection, with expression of lytic cycle antigens, the production of new virus particles and cell death (Sixbey, 1989) In contrast, infection of B lymphocytes leads to activation and immortalization, yielding lymphoblastoid cell lines (LCL) (Pope *et al*, 1969). Resting B cells are induced to enter the cell cycle 48–72 hours after infection, with increased cell size, RNA and DNA synthesis and finally cell division. These changes are accompanied by expression of the cell adhesion molecules and B cell activation antigens, including CD23, which is a marker for EBV immortalization and is shed from the cell surface, acting as an autocrine growth factor for LCL (Swendeman and Thorley-Lawson, 1987). Shortly after infection the linear viral genome circularizes to form an episome in the B cell nucleus and later amplifies to give multiple copies (Hurley and Thorley-Lawson, 1988). A restricted number of viral genes are expressed in LCL—six nuclear antigens (EBNA-1–6) (Dillner and Kallin, 1988), a latent membrane protein (LMP) (Mann and Thorley-Lawson, 1987) and two terminal (membrane) proteins (TP 1 and 2) (Laux *et al*, 1988). This gene expression is termed "latent" and is compatible with continued cell proliferation. It can be induced into a lytic cycle by stimuli that cause B cell differentiation (Crawford and Ando, 1986). The functions of the latent gene products are for the most part unknown, although EBNA-1 maintains the viral episomes in the cell by binding to the origin of replication (Yates *et al*, 1984) and the genes for EBNA-2 and LMP are the putative viral oncogenes. The EBNA-2 deletion mutant P3HRI is non-immortalizing (Dambaugh *et al*, 1986), and the transfection of the EBNA-2 gene into cells infected with P3HRI rescues the immortalization function (Hammerschmidt and Sudgen, 1989). EBNA-2 also transactivates CD23, thereby enhancing autocrine growth (Cordier *et al*, 1990). Latent membrane protein causes a tumorigenic phenotype when transfected into fibroblast cell lines (Wang *et al*, 1985) and upregulates expression of the cell adhesion molecules (Wang *et al*, 1988).

Epstein-Barr Virus Infection In Vivo

Over 90% of adults have evidence of past infection by EBV, primary infection usually occurring asymptomatically during childhood. However, about 50% of individuals whose primary infection is delayed and occurs between the ages of 17 and 25 years experience acute infectious mononucleosis (Niederman *et al*, 1970). Here, the virus enters the body via the mouth and replicates in pharyngeal epithelial cells. From this site B lymphocytes become infected and enter the circulation (Klein *et al*, 1976). Immune mechanisms are stimulated and can be detected at the time of onset of clinical symptoms. These include both cell mediated and humoral responses that control the disease. Large numbers of "atypical" mononuclear cells are seen in the circulation and have been identified as CD8 positive T cells (Crawford *et al*, 1981) with HLA non-restricted cytotoxic activity. These cells are considered essential for recovery from infectious mononucleosis. Serum antibody responses to the virus replicative antigen complexes—viral capsid antigen (VCA), early antigen (EA) and membrane antigen (MA)—appear in a characteristic reaction pattern; IgM antibodies to VCA and a positive heterophil antibody reaction are considered diagnostic of infectious mononucleosis.

Following primary infection, a lifelong carrier state is established, with low grade virus replication in pharyngeal epithelial cells and shedding of infectious virus into the oral cavity (Miller *et al*, 1973). A few circulating B lymphocytes also carry the virus, which, on explantation, give rise to "spontaneous" EBV carrying B cell lines (Nilsson *et al*, 1971). All normal seropositive individuals have IgG antibodies to the VCA and MA complexes which persist for life; the latter neutralize viral infectivity. IgG antibodies to EBNA-1 develop during convalescence from infectious mononucleosis and persist thereafter. Epstein-Barr virus specific memory cytotoxic T cells also appear in the circulation after primary infection and then remain at detectable levels (Rickinson *et al*, 1981). To date, cytotoxic T cell clones specific for the viral antigens EBNA-2 (Moss *et al*, 1988), EBNA-3 (Burrows *et al*, 1990) and LMP (Thorley-Lawson and Israelsohn, 1987) have been demonstrated. These immune mechanisms are thought to control the persistent in vivo infection.

Two theoretical models exist to explain the persistent infection in normal seropositive individuals. The first (Klein, 1989) proposes that long-lived B lymphocytes infected at the time of primary infection are the site of latent infection and are invisible to immune mechanisms because of a very restricted viral gene expression. These cells are triggered into a lytic cycle by local factors while circulating through the oropharynx. The virus produced would be amplified by secondary lytic infection of epithelial cells, which would act as a mode of egress of the virus from the body. An alternative hypothesis (Allday and Crawford, 1988) suggests that latency occurs in the basal epithelial cells of the pharynx, which, as they mature, become permissive for virus replication, with virus release occurring as the mature cells are shed from the epithelial surface. Here B lymphocytes would become infected as they circulate through the lymphoepithelial areas of the pharynx and would be eliminated by immune mechanisms once viral genes are expressed. In both models, the infection would be limited by the action of cytotoxic T cells recognizing specific viral antigens. Positive evidence for this control comes from studies in immuno-suppressed patients where both virus replication in epithelial cells and virus infection of B lymphocytes are increased in parallel with decreased EBV specific cytotoxic T cell activity.

EPSTEIN-BARR VIRUS ASSOCIATED B CELL LYMPHOMA

Burkitt's Lymphoma

Two distinct clinicopathological patterns of BL have been described. Endemic BL (eBL) is prevalent in equatorial Africa and Papua New Guinea. In these areas eBL is the most common childhood tumour, most frequently affecting males and typically giving rise to extranodal tumours that predominantly involve the jaw, gastrointestinal tract and gonads (Lenoir, 1986). The lack of lymph node involvement is a common feature of this tumour. If untreated, eBL is fatal, but it shows a favourable response to cyclophosphamide chemotherapy. Areas of high incidence of BL are found to correlate closely with those where holoendemic malaria occurs, and this has therefore been implicated as a cofactor in the development of the tumour. Evidence of EBV involvement has been found in 96% of BL tumours in endemic areas (Geser *et al*, 1988).

The less common non-endemic or sporadic form of BL (sBL) is reported in economically developed countries but probably has a worldwide distribution. Clinically, sBL shows a bimodal pattern, developing in children older than those associated with eBL and in adults. Like eBL, the principal manifestations of sBL are extranodal, but lymph node involvement has been described. A high proportion of sBL tumours affect the gastrointestinal tract or give rise to primary tumours of the central nervous system (CNS). In contrast to eBL, only 15% of sBL tumours are associated with EBV (Lenoir, 1986). Clinical remissions in sBL can be induced by combination chemotherapy, but the long-term prognosis is poor.

Both types of BL represent clonal proliferations of B cells with restricted immunoglobulin (Ig) expression, usually of IgM type (Pelicci *et al*, 1986). These two types of BL also exhibit chromosomal translocations, which occur at specific breakpoints on chromosome 8 and chromosomes 14, 2 and 22 (Lenoir, 1986). The t(8:14) event is demonstrated in over 90% of BL tumours, and the remaining 10% of tumours are equally affected by the t(8:2) and t(8:22) variants. These genetic alterations appear to be unrelated to the presence or absence of tumour associated EBV.

The chromosomal rearrangements in BL occur at breakpoints in the Ig gene carrying regions on chromosomes 14, 2 or 22 coding for Ig heavy chain (H) and κ and λ light chains, respectively, and within the c-*myc* oncogene region on chromosome 8. Site specific breakpoints appear to correlate with distinct tumour subtypes in that sBL characteristically involves recombination between the switch region of IgH and the c-*myc* gene rather than the JH region typical of eBL (Neri *et al*, 1988). These cytogenetic events are considered to have important relevance to the pathogenesis of BL, since the c-*myc* proto-oncogene in normal cells is pivotal to the control of cell proliferation. Deregulation of c-*myc* arising from the chromosomal translocations in BL results in altered c-*myc* expression and altered cell growth. The nature of the specific breakpoints suggests that in eBL these events take place concurrently with Ig gene rearrangements normally occurring in the early stages of B cell differentiation and in sBL at the stage of isotype switching in a more mature B cell.

The precise role of EBV in the development of a high proportion of eBL is not known. However, in vitro, EBV associated BL cells and BL cell lines show a unique pattern of latent gene product expression. In contrast to the full expression of latent gene products (EBNA-1–6 and LMP) seen in LCL, BL cells in vitro express EBNA-1 alone, implying that EBNA-2 and LMP expression is not necessary for the development of BL.

Large Cell Lymphoma

The increased incidence of large cell lymphoma in iatrogenically immunosuppressed organ transplant recipients has been linked to failure in the control of EBV infection. In 50% of cases, there is evidence of a recent primary EBV infection, whereas the other 50% of tumours arise in individuals who were already seropositive before transplantation. Profound immunosuppression induced by chemotherapeutic agents leads to a well recognized predisposition to the development of certain types of cancer such as NHL, hepatoma and Kaposi's sarcoma. In transplant recipients, the frequency with which these occur is estimated to be 45 to 100 times greater than in the general population. NHL constitutes 26% of all cancers arising in graft recipients and, with the exception of skin and cervical cancers, represents the most frequently occurring tumour group in these patients (Penn, 1983). The risk of postgraft NHL varies with the mode of immunosuppression and type of organ graft. The prevalence of these tumours now appears to be related more to the intensity and prolonged use of combined chemotherapy than to the effects of any one single agent such as cyclosporin. Adoption of careful low dose treatment regimens in recent years has led to a marked reduction in the incidence of postgraft NHL, at least in the context of solid organ grafts (Beveridge *et al*, 1984). In contrast, the recent emergence of lymphoproliferative complications in bone marrow graft recipients may reflect current trends in controlling graft versus host disease and graft rejection by T cell depletion of donor marrow and anti-T cell immunotherapy (Zutter *et al*, 1988).

The clinical presentations of postgraft NHL are characterized by rapid onset, usually within 2 years after transplantation, aggressive behaviour and predilection for extranodal sites. CNS involvement occurs with high frequency in 39-49% of cases (Patchell, 1988) with other frequent sites of presentation in the gastrointestinal tract, lungs and allografted tissue. Although many of these tumours are rapidly fatal, a high proportion of postgraft NHL show an unusual feature of partial or complete regression following reduction or withdrawal of immunosuppressive therapy (Starzl *et al*, 1984). Similar responses have also been reported after treatment with the antiviral agent acyclovir (Hanto *et al*, 1985).

The histopathological patterns of postgraft NHL exhibit striking morphological heterogeneity. The spectrum of changes associated with these lesions is thought to represent different stages in the progression of EBV induced B cell proliferation from diffuse polymorphic B cell hyperplasia to diffuse polymorphic B cell lymphoma (Frizzera, 1981). These patterns are supported by the phenotypic and genotypic heterogeneity of Ig expression exhibited by these tumours. On the basis of cellular Ig phenotyping, the B cell proliferations in postgraft NHL may be polyclonal or monoclonal or may fail to exhibit evidence of detectable Ig synthesis.

Despite phenotypic evidence of polyclonality, in some cases there is increasing evidence that varying proportions of tumour cells in the majority of postgraft NHL contain clonally rearranged Ig gene DNA. Sensitive genotyping studies by Southern blot DNA hybridization have shown that non-clonal and/or clonal populations of proliferating B cells may exist concurrently within single lesions or in several lesions at multiple anatomical sites. The clonal complexity of postgraft NHL is further compounded by evidence that although monoclonal lesions may contain genotypically identical B cells, new Ig gene rearrangements may be present in recurrent lesions at the same site as initial tumour presentation (Hanto *et al,* 1989) or exist as several B cell clones with non-identically rearranged Ig gene DNA either in the same lesion or simultaneously in several lesions at non-contiguous sites. This oligoclonal or multiclonal expression is thought to represent intermediary stages in the progression of hyperplastic B cell populations before the emergence of a single dominant clone. Although karyotyping studies provide evidence of several variable cytogenetic abnormalities in postgraft NHL, none of these lesions have been shown to contain chromosome 8 translocations or c-*myc* rearrangements, which are characteristic of BL.

Evidence of EBV involvement in postgraft NHL has been established by the presence of EBV DNA and expression of EBNA and EBV latent gene products in tumour cell extracts (Saemundsen *et al,* 1982) or localized to tumour cells by various DNA hybridization (Weiss and Movahed, 1989), protein blotting (Thomas *et al,* 1990) and immunocytochemical techniques (Crawford *et al,* 1981). The frequency of EBV related postgraft NHL is estimated at 14% of all cancers developing after transplantation (Touraine *et al,* 1989). Phenotyping studies of postgraft NHL from solid organ and bone marrow transplant recipients show that the patterns of EBV latency in the tumour cells are identical to the EBNA-1, EBNA-2 and LMP profile that characterizes LCLs derived from EBV infected normal B cells in vitro (Thomas *et al,* 1990; Young *et al,* 1989). Furthermore, this pattern is consistent regardless of histological subtype and phenotypic or genotypic expressions of polyclonal, monoclonal or "undetectable" Ig. These observations have considerable significance on the pathogenetic role of EBV in B cell NHL after transplantation. Functional cooperations between EBNA-2 and LMP have several growth potentiating effects on EBV infected B cells in vitro, hence their expression suggests that the virus has a direct oncogenic role in the development of these tumours. EBNA-2 and LMP act as targets for EBV specific cytotoxic T lymphocytes (CTLs) in vitro, and therefore in the normal host, these tumour cells would be recognized and eliminated.

In transplant recipients, profound inhibition of these immunoregulatory T cell controls by drug induced immunosuppression generates a favourable environment for sustained proliferation of B cells with full cellular expression of EBV latent gene products. Tumour cell expression of the B cell activation antigen CD23 (Thomas *et al*, 1990), which is regulated by EBNA-2 and LMP (Wang *et al*, 1988) and also acts as a soluble B cell growth factor (Swendeman and Thorley-Lawson, 1987), may contribute to promoting T cell independent B cell growth in these tumours. The remarkable clinical response of postgraft NHL to reduction or withdrawal of immunosuppression can be attributed to the effects of restoring normal EBV specific immunoregulatory controls, resulting in rapid tumour regression in many of these patients. The mechanism of tumour regression with specific anti-viral therapy remains unclear. However, a significant number of postgraft NHLs are unresponsive to changes in immunosuppression or treatment with antiviral drugs and require more intense forms of combined chemotherapy and radiotherapy. The histological appearances and monoclonal Ig expression in this prognostically poor category suggest that malignant progression has already been established and that manifestations of EBV latency in the tumour cells are irreversibly linked to the malignant process.

NON-HODGKIN LYMPHOMAS IN AIDS

Although NHL may be the presenting symptom of AIDS, it is more frequently the case that HIV seropositive individuals at risk of developing lymphoma have had prior clinical evidence of other AIDS related diseases. Pre-existing diagnosis of AIDS related complex (ARC) particularly with persistent generalized lymphadenopathy, associated opportunistic infections or Kaposi's sarcoma has been reported in 47%, 25% and 11%, respectively, of patients who subsequently developed NHL (Levine *et al*, 1988). Males are more frequently affected than females, and HIV transmission through blood products for haemophilia treatment has been found to be a significant risk factor (Beral *et al*, 1990). AIDS related NHL has a rapidly aggressive clinical pattern and presents as single or multiple tumours with a predilection for extranodal sites. Common sites of presentation are the CNS, gastrointestinal tract and bone marrow. Primary CNS lymphoma was one of the first diagnostic criteria to be recognized for AIDS, since CNS involvement is rare, occurring in approximately 1% of all NHL in non-immunocompromised groups and has been reported recently to constitute about 20% of NHL associated with AIDS (Beral *et al*, 1991). It is now evident that AIDS-NHLs exhibit a wide spectrum of histopathological patterns. The following sections will discuss the high grade BL like and large cell B cell tumours, which are the predominant histological types in AIDS and may be associated with EBV.

"Burkitt's Like Lymphoma" Tumours

A recent study of Centers for Disease Control data shows that BL like lymphomas constitute approximately 20% of AIDS-NHL reported in the USA and have a peak incidence in children and young adults between 10 and 19 years of age (Beral *et al*, 1991). Presentation in the gastrointestinal tract is common, and tumours may show a favourable response to chemotherapy (Kalter *et al*, 1985). Subtypes of AIDS related BL similar to sBL and eBL forms in non-AIDS populations can be distinguished on the basis of cytogenetic abnormalities and involvement with EBV. IgH and c-*myc* switch region translocations were identified in the majority of tumours arising in two independently studied series of AIDS patients with BL like lesions (Pellici *et al*, 1986; Subar *et al*, 1988). Moreover, in both series most of the tumours had no evidence of EBV. These findings are consistent with established cytogenetic and virological patterns of sBL in non-AIDS patient groups. However, in 4 out of 16 patients reported by Subar *et al* (1988) EBV was identified in the tumour cells. Haluska *et al* (1989) have also identified endemic BL like lymphoma associated with t(8:14) and demonstrable EBV DNA carrying tumour cells has also been identified in some AIDS patients. Thus, as shown in Table 1, AIDS related BL appears to exhibit three patterns in which some tumours conform to the EBV negative sBL type, whereas some are more typical of eBL tumours and others are cytogenetically analogous to sBL and are associated with EBV.

"Non-Burkitt's Lymphoma" Tumours

Undifferentiated or immunoblastic lymphoma accounts for 60–80% of reported cases of AIDS-NHL (Levine, 1990; Beral *et al*, 1991) and in older age groups (over 50 years) is more frequently associated with established symptoms of AIDS or ARC (Kalter *et al*, 1985). These tumours are considered to be clinicopathologically similar to the category of B lymphoproliferative neoplasias arising in immunosuppressed organ transplant recipients. Knowles *et al* (1988) have reported three cases of AIDS-NHL with restricted Ig expression that contained EBV DNA but lacked c-*myc*/Ig gene rearrangements. These findings, together with subsequent demonstration of EBV latent gene expression in AIDS related undifferentiated NHL (Thomas and Crawford, 1989), are taken to suggest that EBV has a direct aetiolgical role in these lesions. However, Boiocchi *et al* (1990) have recently identified a subgroup of AIDS-NHL with less obvious viral aetiology. Epstein-Barr virus was demonstrated in one of six cases of NHL developing in patients with intravenously transmitted HIV infection. Furthermore, none of these tumours could be attributed to either the eBL or sBL like category, since typical chromosomal rearrangements were not identified. Clearly, EBV appears not to be essential for the pathogenesis of all non-BL like AIDS lymphomas, suggesting that other factors must be involved.

EPSTEIN-BARR VIRUS AND IMMUNE CONTROL IN AIDS

Imunodeficiency in AIDS Patients

HIV-1 is trophic for cells bearing the CD4 molecule (Dalgleish *et al*, 1984), which are mainly T cells of the helper/inducer subset but also include mono-

TABLE 1. Characteristics of non-Hodgkin lymphoma in AIDS

Tumour group	Chromosomal translocation	EBV genome	Tumour type/ no. of cases	References[a]
BL like tumours	+ (endemic)	+	1 SNCC	1
	+ (sporadic) 1 LC-IBP	+	2 SNCC, 1 LNCC	2
	+ 1 SNCC 1 diffuse LC	+	2 BL type	3, 4, 5
	+ (endemic)	–	3 SNCC	2
	+	–	1 LNCC	
Non-BL tumours	– type 2 LC-IBP	+	3 of uncertain	6, 2, 7
	– 2 LNCC 1 LC-IBP	–	5 SNCC	7, 2

The table summarizes the information available from reports of AIDS NHL, where the presence of chromosomal translocation and EBV genomes have been examined. Endemic, chromosomal translocations characteristic of endemic BL (see text). Sporadic, chromosomal translocations characteristic of sporadic BL, otherwise data not available. SNCC, small non-cleaved cell lymphoma. LC-IBP, large cell immunoblastic plasmacytoid. BL, Burkitt's lymphoma type (all high grade lymphomas). LNCC, large non-cleaved cell (intermediate grade lymphoma).
[a]1 Haluska *et al*, 1989
2 Subar *et al*, 1988
3 Whang-Peng *et al*, 1984
4 Petersen *et al*, 1985
5 Groopman *et al*, 1986
6 Knowles *et al*, 1988
7 Boiocchi *et al*, 1990

cyte-macrophages and Langerhans cells. Infection of these cell types gives individuals infected with the virus a characteristic immunodeficiency. During the course of HIV infection, the number of circulating CD4 positive T cells decreases, causing reversal of the CD4:CD8 ratio. T lymphocytes show a progressive impairment of proliferative responses to mitogens and specific antigens, which may be explained in part by defects in CD4 positive antigen presenting cells and by a direct suppressor effect exerted by the HIV envelope glycoprotein gp120 (Mann *et al*, 1987).

The CD8 positive suppressor/cytotoxic T cell population, although not infected with the virus, has been reported to function abnormally in some instances. In particular, loss of virus specific cytotoxic T cells would appear to correlate with the clinical situation where infections with latent viruses are a constant problem. This may be due to lack of helper/inducer function from the CD4 population. Natural killer cells have also been shown to be defective in AIDS patients. However, in most cases, CD8 positive cytotoxic T cells specific for HIV infected cells can be isolated from the circulation, although their numbers decrease as the disease progresses.

Humoral immunity is also affected in AIDS patients, with polyclonal B cell activation, hypergammaglobulinaemia and impaired B cell responses to T dependent and T independent antigens, all characteristics of HIV infection. Although normal B cells are not infectable by the virus, HIV-1 antigens have been shown to stimulate B cells directly (Clifford-Lane *et al*, 1983), which may in part account for the polyclonal B cell activation seen in these patients. The impaired B cell responses are probably a result of impaired T helper cell function, and this progresses with the disease processes. The consequences of such severe immunodeficiency are a range of uncontrolled opportunistic infections characteristic of AIDS and a greatly increased incidence of tumours, including Kaposi's sarcoma and NHL. The implication of immunodeficiency for EBV replication and infection in NHL are discussed below.

Specific Immune Control of Epstein-Barr Virus Infection in AIDS

In AIDS patients, as in other immunosuppressed individuals, there are many indications that persistent EBV infection is not normally regulated. The fine balance between virus replication and immune control is tipped in favour of virus production, hence levels of EBV replication and shedding from the oropharynx are increased (Alsip *et al*, 1988). Increased levels of IgG antibodies to VCA and a reappearance of anti-EA antibodies may be detected in the early stages of the disease, but these decline as the disease progresses. These changes are presumably all a consequence of a deficient T cell control of the persistent virus infection. Birx *et al* (1986) demonstrated an increased frequency of spontaneously derived B cell lines from peripheral blood of AIDS and ARC patients coincident with a decreased EBV specific T suppressor activity. This decrease in EBV specific immune mechanisms leads to overt disease in many patients. Oral hairy leukoplakia, which is associated with EBV replication in oral mucosal epithelium (Greenspan *et al*, 1985), particularly at the lateral tongue margin in HIV seropositive individuals, has been shown to predict progression to AIDS. Similarly, the incidence of malignant lymphoma in AIDS patients is dramatically increased, and some of these are associated with EBV. However, although it is clear that B cell proliferation predisposes to AIDS-NHL, there is no direct evidence that the B cell proliferation commonly seen in AIDS patients is EBV driven (Crawford *et al*, 1984).

PATHOGENESIS OF NON-HODGKIN LYMPHOMA IN AIDS

The precise aetiology of AIDS-NHL is not known, and on the basis of current available data, it appears that several pathogenetic mechanisms might be involved. That these tumours often develop in the context of reactive lymphoid hyperplasia, as evidenced by the presence of persistent generalized lymphadenopathy or ARC in many patients, suggests that pre-existing B cell hyperproliferation is an important predisposing factor. However, HIV infection per se is unlikely to have a direct role in NHL, since neither the HIV genome nor HIV gene products have been demonstrated in these tumours. It has been suggested that coinfection with other viruses may be necessary for tumour development. Serological evidence of human T lymphotropic virus (HTLV)-I has been reported in some patients with AIDS related B-NHL (Levine *et al*, 1985) and is not uncommon in certain HIV high risk groups (Essex *et al*, 1983). HTLV-I has also been implicated in two cases of B-chronic lymphocytic leukaemia (B-CLL) in which monoclonal Ig synthesized by the leukaemic cells contained specific activity to p24/gp61 structural proteins of the virus (Mann *et al*, 1987). In these cases, HTLV-I was implicated as a source of B cell stimulation, further exacerbated by HTLV-I associated T cell dysfunction, thereby contributing indirectly to the development of malignant B-CLL. The role of these viruses, if any, in causing B cell tumours in AIDS has yet to be substantiated but offers important new areas for further investigation.

The precise role of EBV in AIDS-NHL has not been clarified and may be different in distinct clinicopathological groups. HIV infected individuals usually have normal seropositive profiles or reactivated patterns of persistent EBV infection with increased virus excretion from the oropharynx. This is consistent with HIV induced immunosuppressive effects on normal EBV specific CTLs which regulate persistent infection in vivo. Many BL like tumours in AIDS conform to patterns of classical sBL without evidence of EBV involvement. Other factors yet to be identified, such as other viral agents, are clearly required to produce the oncogenic events that result in malignant B cell growth. EBV infection and c-*myc* activation, which appear to be necessary to produce the tumorigenic phenotype in classical eBL, may also be pertinent to the pathogenesis of EBV associated sBL and the less commonly occurring eBL like tumours in AIDS. This is supported by immunocytochemical (Thomas and Crawford, 1989) and immunoblotting (Allday *et al*, 1990) evidence of restricted EBV latent gene expression in AIDS related BL compatible with the restricted EBNA-1 profile of non-AIDS related BL tumour cells and early passage BL cells in vitro. EBNA-2 expression appears not to be compatible with the development of BL. Failure to express this latent gene product has been suggested to arise from chemical modification of EBV DNA sequences that subsequently inhibits specific gene transcription. CpG methylation of EBNA-2 regulatory gene sequences has recently been identified in BL cell lines in vitro and in tumour cells from AIDS related BL (Allday *et al*, 1990). In contrast, large cell lymphomas in AIDS exhibit full expression of latent gene products, including EBNA-2 and LMP, which attests to the similarity of these tumours with NHL arising with iatrogenic immunosuppression in transplant recipients. The mechanisms for uncontrolled proliferation in these tumours are probably the same as those that produce continued cell growth of EBV infected LCLs in vitro. EBNA-2 and LMP have direct B cell immortalizing functions and may contribute to increased cell proliferation by upregulation of the putative growth factor CD23. Defects in EBV specific CTLs resulting from HIV induced T cell dysfunction lead to failure to control the overwhelming B cell proliferation, resulting in sustained tumour growth. However, EBV is not associated with all tumours of this type. The occurrence of NHL in patients infected with HIV by intravenous routes (where the majority of tumours do not contain EBV) led to the suggestion (Boiocchi *et al*, 1990) that the unusual pathogenic stimuli operating are a result of the different evolution of HIV infection in these patients. This provides yet another alternative for the complex aetiology of these tumours.

SUMMARY

The AIDS-NHLs constitute a histologically diverse group of tumours. Comparisons with some groups of non-AID-NHLs, including eBL, sBL and large cell lymphoma, have been made and similar pathogenetic mechanisms postulated for such groups. However, the incidence of the different pathological types of NHL in AIDS is not yet clear, and further work is necessary to determine the contribution of factors such as c-*myc* translocations and the presence of EBV. AIDS-NHLs are clearly a more diverse group of tumours than their non-AIDS counterparts, and this probably reflects the involvement of a whole range of different pathogenetic stimuli that occur in individual AIDS cases.

References

Allday MJ and Crawford DH (1988) The role of epithelium in EBV persistence and pathogenesis of B cell tumours. *Lancet* **i** 855–858

Allday MJ, Kundu D, Finerty S and Griffin BE (1990) CpG methylation of viral DNA in EBV-associated tumours. *International Journal of Cancer* **45** 1125–1130

Alsip GR, Ench Y, Sumaya CV and Boswell RN (1988) Increased EBV DNA in oropharyngeal secretions from patients with AIDS, AIDS related complex, or asymptomatic human immunodeficiency virus infections. *Journal of Infectious Diseases* **157** 1072–1076

Beral V, Peterman T, Berkelman R and Jaffe H (1991) Non-Hodgkin's lymphoma in persons with AIDS. *Lancet* **337** 805–809

Beveridge T, Krupp P and McKibbin C (1984) Lymphomas and lymphoproliferative lesions developing under cyclosporin therapy. *Lancet* **i** 788

Boiocchi M, Carbone A, De Re V, Dolcetti R, Volpe R and Tivelli V (1990) AIDS related B cell non-Hodgkin's lymphomas in direct blood-stream HIV infected patients: pathogenesis and differentiation features. *International Journal of Cancer* **45** 883–888

Buox DL, Redfield RR and Tosato G (1986) Defective regulation of Epstein-Barr virus infection with acquired immunodeficiency syndrome (AIDS) or AIDS-related disorders. *New England Journal of Medicine* **3** 874–879

Burrows SR, Sculley TB, Misko IS, Schmidt C and Moss DJ (1990) An EBV specific cytotoxic T cell epitope in EBV nuclear antigen 3 (EBNA-3). *Journal of Experimental Medicine* **171** 345–349

Centers for Disease Control (1985) Revision of the case definition of acquired immunodeficiency syndrome for national reporting: United States. *Annals of Internal Medicine* **103** 402–403

Clifford-Lane H, Masur H, Edgar LC, Whalen G, Rook AH and Fauci A (1983) Abnormalities of B-cell activation and immune regulation in patients with the acquired immunodeficiency syndrome. *New England Journal of Medicine* **309** 453–458

Cordier M, Calender A, Billaud M *et al* (1990) Stable transfection of Epstein-Barr virus (EBV) nuclear antigen 2 in lymphoma cells containing the EBV P3HRI genome induces expression of B-cell activation molecules CD21 and CD23. *Journal of Virology* **64** 1002–1013

Crawford DH and Ando I (1986) EB virus induction is associated with B cell maturation. *immunology* **59** 405–409

Crawford DH, Brickell P, Tidman N, McConnel I, Hoffbrand AV and Janossy J (1981) Increased numbers of cells with suppressor T cell phenotype in the peripheral blood of patients with infectious mononucleosis. *Clinical Experimental Immunology* **43** 291–297

Crawford DH, Thomas JA, Janossy G *et al* (1980) Epstein-Barr virus nuclear antigen positive lymphoma after cyclosporin A treatment in a patient with renal allograft. *Lancet* **i** 1355–1356

Crawford DH, Weller I, Iliescu V and Wara DW (1984) Epstein-Barr (EB) virus infection in homosexual men in London. *British Journal of Venereal Diseases* **60** 258–264

Dalgleish AG, Beverley PCL, Clapham PR, Crawford DH, Greaves MF and Weiss RA (1984) The CD4(T4) antigen is an essential component of the receptor for the AIDS retrovirus. *Nature* **312** 763–767

Dambaugh T, Hennessy K, Fennewald S and Kieff E (1986) The viral genome and its expression in latent infection, In: Epstein MA and Achong BG (eds). *The Epstein-Barr Virus: Recent Advances*, pp 14–34, William Heinemann, London

Dillner J and Kalin B (1988) The Epstein-Barr virus proteins. *Advances in Cancer Research* **50** 95–158

Epstein MA (1978) Epstein-Barr virus—discovery, properties and relationship to nasopharyngeal carcinoma, In: de Thé G, Ito Y, and Davis W (eds). *Nasopharyngeal Carcinoma: Aetiology and Control*, pp 333–345, IARC, Lyon

Essex M, McLane MF, Lee TH, Falk L, Howe CWS and Mullins JI (1983) Antibodies to cell membrane antigens associated with T cell leukaemia virus in patients with AIDS. *Science* **220** 859–862

Fingeroth JD, Weiss JJ, Tedder TF, Strominger JL, Biro PA and Fearon DT (1984) Epstein-Barr virus receptor of human B lymphocytes is the C3d receptor CR2. *Proceedings of the National Academy of Sciences of the USA* **81** 4510–4514

Frizzera G, Hanto DW, Gajl-Peczalska KJ *et al* (1981) Polymorphic diffuse B cell hyperplasias and lymphomas in renal transplant recipients. *Cancer Research* **41** 4262–4279

Geser A, Lenoir G, Anvret M *et al* (1988) EBV markers in a series of BLs from the West Nile district, Uganda. *European Journal of Clinical Oncology* **19** 1393–1404

Greenspan JS, Greenspan D, Lennette ET *et al* (1985) Replication of Epstein-Barr virus within the epithelial cells of oral "hairy" leukoplakia, an AIDS-associated lesion. *New England Journal of Medicine* **313** 1564–1571

Grospman JE, Sullivan JL, Mulder C *et al* (1986) Pathogenesis of B-cell lymphoma in a patient with AIDS. *Blood* **67** 612–615

Haluska FC, Russo G, Kant J and Andreef M (1989) Molecular resemblance of an AIDS-associated lymphoma and endemic Burkitt lymphomas: implications of their pathogenesis. *Proceedings of the National Academy of Sciences of the USA* **86** 8907–8911

Hammerschmidt W and Sugden B (1989) Genetic analysis of immortalising functions of Epstein-Barr virus in human B lymphocytes. *Nature* **340** 393–397

Hanto DW, Birkenbach M, Frizzera G, Gijl-Peczalska KJ, Simmons DL and Schubach WH (1989) Confirmation of the heterogeneity of post transplant Epstein-Barr virus-associated B cell proliferations by immunoglobulin gene rearrangement analysis. *Transplantation* **47** 458–464

Hanto DW, Frizzera G, Gajl-Peczalska KJ and Simmons RL (1985) Epstein-Barr virus, immunodeficiency and B cell lymphoproliferation. *Transplantation* **39** 461–472

Henle G, Henle W and Diehl V (1968) Relation of Burkitt's tumour-associated herpes-type virus to infectious mononucleosis. *Proceedings of the National Academy of Sciences of the USA* **59** 94–101

Hotchin NA, Thomas JA, Allday MJ *et al* (1990) Immunohistology of Epstein-Barr virus-associated antigens in B cell disorders from individuals. *Transplantation* 49 944–953D

Hurley EA and Thorley-Lawson DA (1988) B cell activation and the establishment of Epstein-Barr virus latency. *Journal of Experimental Medicine* 186 2059–2075

Kalter SP, Riggs SA, Cabanillas F *et al* (1985) Aggressive non-Hodgkin's lymphomas in immunocompromised homosexual males. *Blood* 66 655–659

Klein G, Svedmyr E, Jondal M and Persson PO (1976) EBV determined nuclear antigen (EBNA)-positive cells in the peripheral blood of infectious mononucleosis patient. *International Journal of Cancer* 17 21–26

Klein G (1989) Viral latency and transformation: The strategy of Epstein-Barr virus. *Cell* 58 5–8

Knowles DM, Chamulak GA, Subar M *et al* (1988) Lymphoid neoplasia associated with the acquired immunodeficiency syndrome (AIDS). *Annals of Internal Medicine* 108 744–753

Laux G, Perricaudet M and Farrell P (1988) A spliced Epstein-Barr virus gene expressed in immortalised lymphocytes is created by circularisation of the linear viral genome. *EMBO Journal* 7 769–774

Lenoir GM (1986) Role of the virus chromosomal translocation and cellular oncogenes in the aetiology of Burkitt's lymphoma, In: Epstein MA and Achong BG (eds). *The Epstein Barr Virus: Recent Advances,* p 183, William Heinemann, London

Levine, AM (1988) Reactive and neoplastic lymphoproliferative disorders and other miscellaneous cancers associated with HIV infection, In: Devita VT, Hellman S and Rosenberg SA (eds). *AIDS. Aetiology, Diagnosis, Treatment and Prevention*, pp 263–275, Lippincott, Philadelphia

Levine AM (1990) Lymphoma in acquired immunodeficiency syndrome. *Seminars in Oncology* 17 104–112

Levine AM, Gill PS, Meyer PR, Burkes RL, Ross R, Dworsky RD, Krailo M, Parker JW, Lukes RJ and Rasheed S (1985) Retrovirus and malignant lymphoma in homosexual men. *Journal of the Americal Medical Association* 254 1921–1925

Lowenthal DA, Straus DJ, Wise Campbell S, Gold JEM, Clarkson BD and Koziner B (1988) AIDS-related lymphoid neoplasia: the Memorial Hospital experience. *Cancer* 61 2325–2337

Mann DL, Lasane F, Dopovic M *et al* (1987) HTLV-III large envelope protein (gp120) suppresses PHA-induced lymphocyte blastogenesis. *Journal of Immunology* 138 2640

Mann KP and Thorley-Lawson D (1987) Post translational processing of the Epstein Barr virus-encoded p63/LMP protein. *Journal of Virology* 61 2100–2108

Miller G, Niederman JC and Andrews LL (1973) Prolonged oropharyngeal excretion of Epstein-Barr virus after infectious mononucleosis. *New England Journal of Medicine* 288 229–232

Moss DJ, Misko IS, Burrows SR, Burman K, McCarthy R and Sculley TB (1988) Cytotoxic T-cell clones discriminate between A and B type Epstein Barr virus transformants. *Nature* 331 719–721

Moss DJ, Rickinson AB, Wallace LE and Epstein MA (1981) Sequential appearance of Epstein-Barr virus nuclear and lymphocyte-detected membrane antigens in B cell transformation. *Nature* 291 664–666

Neri A, Barriga, F, Knowles DM, Magrath IT and Dalla-Favera R (1988) Different regions of the Ig heavy chain locus are involved in chromosomal translocations in distinct pathogenic forms of BL. *Proceedings of the National Academy of Sciences of the USA* 85 2748

Niederman JC, Evans AS, Subrahmanyan L and McCollum RW (1970) Prevalence, incidence and persistence of EB virus antibody in young adults. *New England Journal of Medicine* 282 361–365

Nilsson K, Klein G, Henle W and Henle G (1971) The establishment of lymphoblastoid cell lines from adult and fetal human lymphoid tissue and its dependence on EBV. *International Journal of Cancer* 8 443–450

Patchell RA (1988) Primary central nervous system lymphoma in the transplant patient.

Neurologic Clinics **6** 297–303

Pattengale PL, Smith RW and Gerber P (1973) Selective transformation of B lymphocytes by EB virus. *Lancet* **ii** 93–94

Pelicci PG, Knowles DM, Magrath I and Dalla-Favera R (1986) Chromosomal breakpoints and structural rearrangements of the c-*myc* locus differ in endemic and sporadic forms of Burkitt's lymphoma. *Proceedings of the National Academy of Sciences of the USA* **83** 2984–2988

Penn I (1983) Lymphomas complicating organ transplantation. *Transplantation Proceedings* **15** (4) (Suppl) 2790–2797

Peterson JM, Tubbs RR, Savage RA *et al* (1985) Small noncleaved B cell Burkitt-like lymphoma with chromosome t(8;14) translocation and Epstein-Barr virus nuclear-associated antigen in a homosexual man with acquired immune deficiency syndrome. *Americal Journal of Medicine* **78** 141–148

Pope JH, Horne MK and Scott W (1969) Identification of the filtrable leucocyte-transforming factor of QIMR-WIL cells as a herpes-like virus. *International Journal of Cancer* **4** 255–260

Rickinson AB, Moss DJ and Wallace LE (1981) Longterm T-cell mediated immunity to Epstein Barr virus. *Cancer Research* **41 (Supplement)** 4216–4221

Saemundsen AK, Klein G, Cleary M and Warnke R (1982) Epstein-Barr virus carrying lymphoma in cardiac transplant recipient. *Lancet* **i** 158

Sixbey JW (1989) Epstein Barr virus and epithelial cells. *Advances in Viral Oncology* **8** 187–202

Sixbey JW, Davis DS, Young LS *et al* (1987) Human epithelial cell expression of an Epstein-Barr virus receptor. *Journal of General Virology* **68** 805–811

Sixbey JW, Nedrud JG, Raab-Truab N, Hanes RA and Pagano JS (1984) Epstein-Barr virus replication in oropharyngeal epithelial cells. *New England Journal of Medicine* **310** 1225–1230

Starzl TF, Porter KA, Iwatsuki S *et al* (1984) Reversibility of lymphomas or lymphoproliferative lesions developing under cyclosporin-steroid therapy. *Lancet* **i** 583–587

Subar M, Neri A, Inghirami G, Knowles DM and Dalla-Favera R (1988) Frequent c-*myc* oncogene activation and infrequent presence of Epstein-Barr virus genome in AIDS associated lymphoma. *Blood* **72** 667–671

Swendeman S and Thorley-Lawson DA (1987) The activation antigen Blast-2, when shed, is an autocrine BCGF for normal and transformed B cells. *EMBO Journal* **6** 1637–1642

Thomas JA and Crawford DH (1989) EBV associated B cell lymphoma in AIDS and after organ transplantation. *Lancet* **i** 1075–1076

Thorley-Lawson DA and Israelsohn ES (1987) Generation of specific cytotoxic T cells with a fragment of the Epstein Barr virus encoded p63/latent membrane protein. *Proceedings of the National Academy of Sciences of the USA* **84** 5384–8388

Touraine JL, Garnier JL, Lefrancois N *et al* (1989) Severe lymphoproliferative disease and Kaposi's sarcoma in transplant patients. *Transplantation Proceedings* **21** 3179–3198

Wang D, Liebowitz D and Kieff E (1985) An EBV membrane protein expressed in immortalised lymphocytes transforms established rodent cells. *Cell* **43** 831–840

Wang D, Liebowitz D, Wang F *et al* (1988) Epstein-Barr virus latent infection membrane protein alters the human B-lymphocyte phenotype: deletion of the amino terminus abolishes activity. *Journal of Virology* **62** 4173–4184

Weiss LM and Movahed LA (1989) In situ demonstration of Epstein-Barr viral genomes in viral-associated B lymphoproliferation. *Americal Journal of Pathology* **134** 651–659

Whang-Peng J, Lee EL, Sievents H and Magrath IT (1984) Burkitts lymphoma in AIDS: Cytogenetic study. *Blood* **63** 818–822

Yates J, Warren N, Reisman D and Sugden B (1984) A cis-acting element from the EB viral genome that permits stable replication of recombinant plasmids in latently infected cells. *Proceedings of the National Academy of Sciences of the USA* **81** 3806–3810

Young L, Alfieri C, Hennessy K *et al* (1989) Expression of Epstein-Barr virus transformation-associated genes in tissues of patients with EBV lymphoproliferative disease. *New England*

Journal of Medicine **321** 1080–1085

Ziegler JL, Miner RC, Rosenbaum E *et al* (1982) Outbreak of Burkitt's-like Lymphoma in homosexual men. *Lancet* **ii** 631–633

Ziegler JI, Beckstead JA, Volberding PA *et al* (1984) Non-Hodgkin's lymphoma in 90 homosexual men: relation to generalised lymphadenopathy and the acquired immunodeficiency syndrome. *New England Journal of Medicine* **311** 565–570.

Zutter MM, Martin PJ, Sale GE, Shulman HM, Fisher L, Thomas ED and Durnam DM (1988) EBV lymphoproliferation after bone marrow transplantation. *Blood* **72** 520–529.

The authors are responsible for the accuracy of the references.

Clinical Manifestations and Treatment of HIV Related Non-Hodgkin Lymphoma

Donald W Northfelt[1] • Lawrence D Kaplan[2]

[1]Division of AIDS Activities/Oncology, University of California, San Francisco, California;
[2]San Francisco General Hospital, San Francisco, California 94110

INTRODUCTION

The association of malignant lymphoma with AIDS has been recognized since early in the current epidemic (Ziegler *et al*, 1982; Centers for Disease Control, 1982). Recognition of this association led to the inclusion of non-Hodgkin lymphoma (NHL) in the revised case definition of AIDS developed by the US Centers for Disease Control in 1985 (Centers for Disease Control, 1985). AIDS related NHL (AIDS-NHL) has clinical manifestations analogous to malignant lymphoma arising in other acquired (Hanto *et al*, 1981; Penn, 1983) and congenital (Purtilo, 1980) immunodeficiency states. Thus the presentation of AIDS-NHL consists primarily of tumours with B cell phenotype, intermediate or high grade histological subtype and rapid clinical progression. There is a high frequency of unusual extranodal involvement, including a propensity for involvement of the central nervous system (CNS) and bone marrow. Therapy for AIDS-NHL has been largely unsatisfactory, with responses to standard treatments being both less frequent and less durable than in comparable patients without AIDS.

It has been suggested that the incidence of AIDS-NHL is likely to increase significantly as physicians become more adept at suppressing and treating the infectious sequelae of HIV infection (Pluda *et al*, 1990). Understanding of the basic biology, clinical presentation and treatment of AIDS-NHL will therefore become increasingly important in the medical management of patients with AIDS as the second decade of the epidemic commences. This chapter will review features of the clinical presentation and treatment of AIDS-NHL.

CLINICAL PRESENTATION

Patient Characteristics

Unlike the other common HIV related malignancy, Kaposi's sarcoma, which occurs almost exclusively in homosexual men (Beral *et al*, 1990), AIDS-NHL has been reported in all groups at risk for HIV infection. Early reports described malignant lymphoma only in homosexual men (Centers for Disease Control, 1982; Ziegler *et al*, 1982, 1984; Kalter *et al*, 1985; Levine *et al*, 1985), but in subsequent reports, the development of AIDS-NHL has also been noted in intravenous drug users, transfusion recipients and heterosexual contacts (Italian Cooperative Group for AIDS-related Tumours, 1988; Knowles *et al*, 1988; Lowenthal *et al*, 1988; Kaplan *et al*, 1989a). No differences have been reported among the various risk groups with respect to clinical manifestations of AIDS-NHL or response to therapy.

At present, NHL is the index AIDS diagnosis in approximately 3% of new cases of AIDS (Centers for Disease Control, 1990). However, some preliminary data and recent experience at San Francisco General Hospital (SFGH) suggest that AIDS-NHL is becoming a more frequent AIDS defining illness in persons with HIV infection. Kaplan *et al* (1989a) noted retrospectively that the incidence of AIDS-NHL as an index AIDS diagnosis rose from 2.5% in 1985 to 5.0% in 1987 at SFGH. The corresponding figure for 1990 is 8%. A further suggestion of this trend is found in data from a prospective study of pulmonary complications of HIV infection which has enrolled 253 seropositive subjects without AIDS in San Francisco. AIDS developed in 28 subjects from this cohort during 6 to 20 months of follow-up, and in 4 (14%) of these, AIDS-NHL was the AIDS defining illness (Hopewell P., personal communication). Data such as these lend support to speculation that improvements in prevention and treatment of opportunistic infections, and in treatment for HIV infection itself, may be reducing mortality from other causes and thereby increasing the population at risk for developing AIDS-NHL (Freter, 1990; Pluda *et al*, 1990).

Primary CNS lymphoma in AIDS appears to differ from peripheral AIDS-NHL, ie AIDS-NHL outside the CNS, with respect to HIV related disease status at presentation. For example, of the 80 patients with peripheral AIDS-NHL seen at SFGH between October 1981 and May 1988, only 24 of 80 (30%) had a diagnosis of AIDS before the development of lymphoma (Kaplan *et al*, 1989a). In contrast, AIDS had been previously diagnosed in 46 of 55 (84%) cases of primary CNS AIDS-NHL diagnosed in San Francisco between

March 1982 and February 1989 (Baumgartner *et al*, 1990). This suggests that primary CNS AIDS-NHL develops as a consequence of more profound or prolonged immunodeficiency. The recent report by Pluda *et al* (1990) lends further support to this concept; they noted the development of AIDS-NHL in 8 patients from a cohort of 55 patients with prolonged severe immunodeficiency who had been followed prospectively for an average of 23.8 months while receiving various anti-retroviral therapies. Four of the eight patients in this group (50%) developed primary CNS AIDS-NHL, a considerably higher proportion than the 17% (58 of 328) with primary CNS AIDS-NHL found within the four largest series reported in the literature (Ziegler *et al*, 1984; Italian Cooperative Group for AIDS-related Tumours, 1988; Knowles *et al*, 1988; Kaplan *et al*, 1989a). No firm conclusions should be drawn from comparison of disparate sets of retrospective data such as these, but this information does coincide with our clinical impression that primary CNS AIDS-NHL is usually associated with severe immunodeficiency and end stage HIV infection.

Presenting Clinical Features

The clinical presentation of AIDS-NHL is characterized by widespread disease at diagnosis, with frequent involvement of extranodal sites. In the series reported by Ziegler *et al* (1984) 95% of patients had evidence of extranodal disease at presentation, including 42% with some involvement of the nervous system and 33% with bone marrow involvement. Extranodal lymphoma was present in 87% and 65% of patients in two other large series (Knowles *et al*, 1988; Lowenthal *et al*, 1988). The most common sites of disease in these series included the gastrointestinal tract, nervous system (brain or meninges), bone marrow, liver and lung. In the SFGH series, 67% of the patients presented with stage IV disease, including 43% in whom extranodal disease was present (Table 1) and 31% in whom there was no identifiable site of nodal disease (Kaplan *et al*, 1989a).

As has been observed in other immunosuppressed patients with NHL, unusual extralymphatic presentations are common. AIDS related NHL has been found in the rectum (Burkes *et al*, 1986), heart and pericardium (Balasubramanyam *et al*, 1986; Guarner *et al*, 1987) and common bile duct (Kaplan *et al*, 1989b). Gastrointestinal involvement has been reported in up to 27% of patients with AIDS-NHL (Friedman, 1988) with lymphoma being found in virtually any site in the hollow viscera and hepatobiliary tree. Other unusual sites of disease in the SFGH series included subcutaneous and soft tissue, the epidural space, appendix, gingiva, parotid gland and paranasal sinuses (Kaplan *et al*, 1989a).

Because of the highly variable anatomical distribution of AIDS-NHL, it is difficult to make generally applicable statements regarding the clinical presentation of the disease. In our experience, however, there are certain clinical settings in which the diagnosis of lymphoma should be strongly considered (Table 2). Rapid enlargement of a lymph node or group of nodes probably

TABLE 1. Sites of extranodal AIDS NHL in 62 patients at San Francisco General Hospital

Site	No. of patients
Bone marrow	26
Liver	22
Meninges	10
Lung	5
Soft tissue	4
Brain	4
Rectum	3
Epidural	3
Stomach	1
Small bowel	1
Appendix	1
Bile duct	1
Testis	1
Pericardium	1
Gingiva	1
Parotid gland	1

constitutes the most common presenting feature of AIDS-NHL, despite the frequency of extranodal disease described above. Rapidly enlarging lymphadenopathy in a patient with HIV infection should therefore lead to an aggressive evaluation for the presence of lymphoma. This situation must be distinguished from the persistent generalized lymphadenopathy found in many such patients. Careful history taking and documentation of lymph node status on routine examinations can aid in making this distinction. The possibility of lymphoma should also be considered when a mass develops in the pharynx or tonsillar region. Delay in diagnosis can result when such findings are ascribed to abscess formation. AIDS related NHL should be suspected when one or multiple pulmonary nodules are seen to enlarge on serial radiographs; we and others (Polish et al, 1989) have seen several such cases in which the diagnosis was obscure until the patient came to necropsy. Anorectal lymphoma is another manifestation of AIDS-NHL that requires special consideration. Homosexual men are prone to the development of various forms of anorectal disease, including fissures, fistulae, abscesses and condylomata. In several patients at SFGH, anorectal lymphomas were discovered after standard thera-

TABLE 2. Common clinical settings in which the diagnosis of AIDS NHL must be strongly considered

Rapidly enlarging lymph node or nodal group
Enlarging mass in the upper respiratory and digestive tracts
Pulmonary mass or nodule
Rectal mass
Brain mass
Multiple cranial neuropathies

pies for other conditions had failed. Other manifestations of gastrointestinal lymphoma include abdominal pain, symptoms of obstruction and bleeding.

Patients with AIDS-NHL occasionally complain only of constitutional symptoms such as weight loss, fatigue and fever. Although a number of HIV related opportunistic infections, and HIV infection itself, frequently cause similar symptoms, a careful physical examination and screening laboratory investigations (serum lactate dehydrogenase, chest radiograph, gallium isotopic scan) can be useful in clarifying the diagnosis.

Meningeal lymphoma commonly occurs in association with disease at other nodal or extranodal sites, but when lymphoma occurs within the brain in HIV infected patients, there is usually no disease at other sites. Headache and multiple cranial neuropathies are the most common presenting features of meningeal lymphoma (Levine *et al*, 1985). Confusion, memory loss, lethargy, hemiparesis, dysphasia and seizures are the signs and symptoms seen most frequently with primary CNS AIDS-NHL (Baumgartner *et al*, 1990).

DIAGNOSIS

Histopathological or cytological examination is necessary to confirm the diagnosis of AIDS-NHL, and early pathological examination can help to distinguish lymphoma from a number of other conditions that present in similar ways. As noted above, many patients with HIV infection have chronic reactive lymphadenopathy, which can be confused with malignant disease. Kaposi's sarcoma can involve lymph nodes, causing massive enlargement. Mycobacteria, *Pneumocystis carinii*, cat-scratch bacillus and other infectious agents may produce lymphadenopathy, organomegaly and mass lesions that are clinically indistinguishable from those caused by lymphoma.

Imaging studies of the chest, abdomen and pelvis must be performed to fully define the extent of lymphomatous involvement (Nyberg *et al*, 1986). In this way, specific disease related complications such as ureteral or biliary obstruction, impingement on airways and vascular structures and impending or actual compression of nerve roots or the spinal cord can be identified. In addition, these studies provide a baseline for later comparison to assess the benefit of therapy. Bone marrow biopsy and lumbar puncture for spinal fluid cytology are performed for similar reasons.

The clinical presentation and radiographic findings associated with primary CNS AIDS-NHL are sometimes difficult to distinguish from those produced by cerebral toxoplasmosis. Patients presenting with suspicious neurological symptoms should have prompt evaluation with computed tomographic (CT) or magnetic resonance (MR) scan of the brain. Ciricillo and Rosenbaum (1990) recently reported on the use of MR scan to distinguish between toxoplasmosis and lymphoma. In their series, 12 of 17 solitary lesions seen on MR scan were eventually determined to be lymphoma. In contrast, among 35 patients with multiple lesions, 12 were found to be lymphoma and 9 were toxoplasmosis.

Gill *et al* (1985) also found that CNS AIDS-NHL is also more likely to present as a solitary lesion on imaging studies.

However, in current clinical practice the results of CT or MR scan are rarely relied upon to determine the specific aetiology of a mass lesion in the brain. Instead, if focal lesions are demonstrated on imaging studies of the brain, a serum specimen should be sent for toxoplasma titres. Since toxoplasmosis is rare in individuals with negative toxoplasma serologies (Navia *et al*, 1986), brain biopsy should be performed in a timely fashion in this group of patients. Individuals with focal intracerebral lesions and positive serology for toxoplasma are typically started on anti-toxoplasma therapy and observed closely for signs of improvement or deterioration. If there is no improvement in symptoms or findings on repeat imaging studies after 10–14 days of therapy, a brain biopsy should be performed to establish the diagnosis histologically.

TREATMENT

Retrospective Studies

Multiagent chemotherapeutic regimens have been developed for the treatment of intermediate and high grade NHLs in non-HIV infected individuals. Treatment with these regimens has resulted in a dramatic improvement in prognosis for such patients (DeVita *et al*, 1988). Complete responses in up to 86% of cases, and long-term survival in up to 65% of cases, have been reported in patients treated for aggressive large cell lymphomas with these regimens (Connors and Klimo, 1988).

Patients with AIDS-NHL have been treated with standard combination chemotherapy regimens known to be effective against aggressive lymphomas. Unfortunately, the results of such therapies in AIDS-NHL patients have been much less rewarding than the results seen in non-HIV infected individuals. Complete response rates are lower than the corresponding rates seen in the non-HIV infected population, and responses that do occur tend to be of short duration. These general observations were derived from retrospective studies (Table 3) describing patients with AIDS-NHL treated with standard chemotherapy regimens, including CHOP (cyclophosphamide adriomycin oncovin

TABLE 3. Response to chemotherapy in retrospective studies of AIDS NHL

Reference	No. of patients	Complete response (%)
Knowles *et al*, 1988	83	33
Ziegler *et al*, 1984	66	53
Kaplan *et al*, 1989	65	54
Lowenthal *et al*, 1988	30	56
Italian Cooperative Group, 1988	26	35
Bermudez *et al*, 1988	12	17

[vincristine] prednisolone), CVP (cyclophosphamide vincristine prednisolone), M-BACOD (methotrexate bleomycin adriomycin cyclophosphamide oncovin dexamethasone), MACOP-B (methotrexate adriomycin cyclophosphamide oncovin prednisolone bleomycin) and others at a number of institutions. Duration of complete response to chemotherapy and median survival time of chemotherapy treated patients in these studies ranged from 4 to 6 months. Deaths were most frequently due to recurrent lymphoma or opportunistic infections. Several authors noted that the AIDS-NHL patients had poor bone marrow reserve resulting in more severe chemotherapy induced cytopenias than would usually be expected with such therapy (Gill *et al*, 1987; Bermudez *et al*, 1989; Kaplan *et al*, 1989a).

Important prognostic information has been obtained from retrospective studies of therapy for AIDS-NHL. Investigators from New York University reported that the morphological subtype of lymphoma may predict response to therapy (Knowles *et al*, 1988). They obtained complete responses in 52% of patients with AIDS-NHL and large non-cleaved cell histology; the comparable figure for small non-cleaved cell and immunoblastic histologies were 26% and 21%, respectively. Morphological subtype was also predictive of survival in this series. Patients with intermediate grade large cell lymphoma had the longest median survival time (7.5 months), whereas those with small non-cleaved cell lymphoma had a median survival time of 5.5 months, and those with immunoblastic lymphoma had a median survival time of only 2.0 months.

In the SFGH series (Kaplan *et al*, 1989a) median survival time for all patients with AIDS-NHL receiving chemotherapy was 5.5 months. However, clinical features were identified within this cohort that were associated with longer survival (Table 4). Those features identified as being predictive of significantly improved survival included an absolute CD4+ lymphocyte count above 100 cells/µl, absence of a prior AIDS diagnosis, Karnofsky performance

TABLE 4. Median survival associated with specific clinical features in AIDS NHL

Clinical feature	Median survival months	p-value for difference
CD4 lymphocyte count		
<100 cells/µl	4.1	
>100 cells/µl	24	0.01
Prior AIDS diagnosis		
yes	2.2	
no	8.3	0.0001
Karnofsky performance status		
<70%	3.8	
≥70%	6.8	0.03
Extranodal disease		
present	4.2	
absent	12.2	0.01

score ≥70% and the absence of an extranodal site of disease. Evaluation of these prognostic features may be of assistance in determining how to approach therapy in newly diagnosed patients. Data from the same study also suggested that treatment of AIDS-NHL with less aggressive chemotherapy may result in better response or longer survival. Patients who received ≥1 g/m² cyclophosphamide per treatment cycle had a median survival time of only 4.6 months, whereas those receiving <1 g/m² cyclophosphamide per treatment cycle had a median survival time of 12.2 months.

Prospective Studies

A number of prospective studies of chemotherapy for AIDS-NHL have also been undertaken. The first, reported by Gill *et al* (1987), consisted of two sequential phase II studies. The initial group of 13 patients received the standard M-BACOD regimen. The second group was treated with a novel regimen consisting of induction therapy with high dose cytosine arabinoside, L-asparaginase, vincristine, prednisone, cyclophosphamide (1.5 g/m²) and high dose methotrexate with leucovorin rescue, followed with consolidation therapy with three cycles of CHOP alternating with three cycles of etoposide given every 21 days. Central nervous system prophylaxis with 2400 cGy radiotherapy to a helmet field was given to patients in the second group. Complete responses occurred in 54% of patients in the M-BACOD group, with 31% achieving more than 1 year disease free survival; CNS (meningeal) progression occurred in 15%. In contrast, only 33% of patients who received the novel regimen obtained a complete response: 11% achieved over 1 year disease free survival, and 67% developed progressive disease in the CNS. Median survival time for the M-BACOD group was 11 months, versus 6 months in the patients who received the novel regimen. The investigators concluded that the novel intensive regimen was associated with a significant risk of early death due to opportunistic infection and hematological toxicity; they therefore suggested that less intensive treatment strategies be explored. Furthermore, the frequency of meningeal progression or relapse in their patients indicated the need for early incorporation of CNS prophylaxis in treatment strategies for AIDS-NHL.

As part of a larger study detailing the clinical characteristics of patients with AIDS-NHL at SFGH, Kaplan *et al* (1989) reported on the treatment of 38 patients in a prospective chemotherapy trial. A regimen (COMET-A) was devised that consisted of cyclophosphamide (1.4 g/m²), vincristine, methotrexate with leucovorin rescue, etoposide and cytarabine. Patients also received CNS prophylaxis with four intrathecal injections of methotrexate and monthly pneumocystis prophylaxis with intravenous pentamidine (4 mg/kg/month). Complete responses were seen in 58% of patients treated with COMET-A, a proportion that was not statistically different from the 46% of patients with complete responses in a historical control group treated with a variety of standard regimens. In addition, the median survival time of the

COMET-A group (5.2 months) was significantly shorter than that of the controls (11.3 months).

The results of these studies led investigators to conclude that dose intensive myelosuppressive chemotherapy regimens containing high dose cyclophosphamide resulted in shortened survival in patients with AIDS-NHL. As a consequence of this experience, a prospective multicentre clinical trial was performed to evaluate the efficacy of lower dose chemotherapy for AIDS-NHL (Levine *et al*, 1989). In this regimen, a modification of the standard M-BACOD protocol was employed in which the cyclophosphamide dose was reduced from 600 to 300 mg/m^2/cycle, and the doxorubicin dose was reduced from 45 to 25 mg/m^2/cycle. Prophylaxis for meningeal lymphoma and pneumocystis pneumonia was required. Fifteen of 35 patients (43%) who could be evaluted achieved complete responses, and 10 of the complete responders remained in continuous complete remission from 7+ to 26+ months from discontinuation of chemotherapy.

Another approach to ameliorating the toxicities of chemotherapy in patients with AIDS-NHL has recently been described by Kaplan *et al* (1991). They carried out a prospective randomized trial to determine whether recombinant human granulocyte-macrophage colony stimulating factor (rGM-CSF) would reduce chemotherapy induced myelosuppression and its sequelae. In this study, treatment consisted of CHOP chemotherapy accompanied by prophylaxis for meningeal lymphoma and pneumocystis pneumonia. Patients receiving rGM-CSF on days 4–13 of each 21 day treatment cycle had significantly higher absolute neutrophil counts at chemotherapy induced nadir, shorter mean duration of neutropenia, fewer chemotherapy cycles complicated by neutropenia and fever and fewer days in hospital for neutropenia and fever compared with patients who received no rGM-CSF. Complete responses were observed in 67% of control patients and 70% of rGM-CSF treated patients, with median survival times of 9.0 and 11.4 months, respectively. However, the response and survival data must be interpreted with caution, because patients enrolled in this study were generally healthier than what would be expected for an unselected population of patients with AIDS-NHL.

Bone marrow transplantation is an effective therapy for patients with NHL who have a poor prognosis (Appelbaum *et al*, 1987). A recent report described the use of this approach in a patient with AIDS-NHL (Holland *et al*, 1989). A 41 year old HIV infected man with AIDS-NHL involving the liver and meninges was treated with M-BACOD as induction therapy, followed by high dose cyclophosphamide, intravenous zidovudine, total body irradiation and allogeneic bone marrow donated by his HLA compatible sister. Engraftment of donor marrow was documented, but the lymphoma recurred 39 days after the transplant, and the patient died 8 days later. At necropsy, no evidence of persistent HIV genetic material was found in analysis of a number of tissues by polymerase chain reaction gene amplification. The authors concluded that this strategy might eradicate HIV infection, although it was ineffective as therapy for the lymphoma in this case.

Treatment of Primary CNS Lymphoma in AIDS

There have been no prospective studies of therapy for primary CNS AIDS-NHL. Most retrospective studies and case reports published to date have described the use of radiation therapy as primary treatment for CNS AIDS-NHL. Formenti *et al* (1989) reported that whole brain irradiation, in doses ranging from 2200 to 5000 cGy and combined with partial tumour resection and systemic chemotherapy in some cases, resulted in complete responses in six of ten patients. Median survival time for the group was 5.5 months, and half of the patients died of opportunistic infections. Baumgartner *et al* (1990) reported the results of treatment in 29 patients with CNS AIDS-NHL. The therapy consisted of irradiation with 2130 to 5400 cGy using various fractionation schemes; a small number of patients also underwent partial tumour resections and/or received systemic chemotherapy. The median survival time for this group was 4 months. A group of 26 other patients who received no treatment had a median survival time of 1 month. Similar results have been reported by other investigators (Gill *et al*, 1985; So *et al*, 1986; Remick *et al*, 1990). In all of these studies, most patients have died of opportunistic infections. Therefore, development of more effective therapy for primary CNS AIDS-NHL may require improvements in the treatment of HIV associated opportunistic infections.

Current Treatment Approaches

Experience in the treatment of AIDS-NHL to date suggests that therapies designed to cause less myelosuppression used in conjunction with aggressive efforts to prevent opportunistic infections are needed. Such strategies form the basis of a study currently being conducted by the AIDS Clinical Trials Group (ACTG) of the US National Institutes of Health. Patients entering this study are randomized to receive either the low dose M-BACOD regimen previously tested by the ACTG (Levine *et al*, 1989) or standard dose M-BACOD in combination with rGM-CSF to ameliorate chemotherapy induced myelotoxicity. All patients receive monthly aerosolized pentamidine as pneumocystis prophylaxis. The results of this study will help to clarify the relative merits and drawbacks of dose intensive versus marrow sparing therapy.

CONCLUSION

The incidence of AIDS-NHL may increase as therapy for and prevention of other complications of HIV infection improve. AIDS related NHL has remained one of the most difficult problems faced by physicians treating patients with HIV infection, despite the knowledge and experience that has been acquired in the course of the epidemic. The clinical presentation of the disease is extremely variable and often diagnostically challenging. Less aggressive therapy appears to be more tolerable to patients with AIDS-NHL, but the efficacy of current therapies remains unsatisfactory. It is hoped that future advances in understanding the basic biology of lymphoma and HIV related immunodeficiency will lead to improvements in treatment of AIDS-NHL.

SUMMARY

Non-Hodgkin lymphoma developing in patients with HIV infection fulfills diagnostic criteria for AIDS. Clinical manifestations of AIDS-NHL are similar to those of malignant lymphoma arising in other acquired and congenital immunodeficiency states. AIDS related NHLs therefore consist primarily of tumours with B cell phenotype, intermediate or high grade histological subtype and rapid clinical progression with a high frequency of unusual extranodal involvement. Treatment of AIDS-NHL has been much less rewarding than treatment of lymphoma in non-HIV infected individuals. Complete response rates are lower than the corresponding rates seen in the non-HIV infected population, and responses that do occur tend to be of short duration. Improvements in treatment for AIDS-NHL will require the use of new therapies, designed to cause less myelosuppression, in conjunction with aggressive efforts to prevent opportunistic infections.

References

Applebaum FR, Sullivan KM, Buckner CD *et al* (1987) Treatment of malignant lymphoma in patients with chemotherapy, total body irradiation, and bone marrow transplantation. *Journal of Clinical Oncology* **5** 1340–1347

Balasubramanyan A, Waxman M, Kazal HL and Lee MH (1986) Malignant lymphoma of the heart in acquired immunodeficiency syndrome. *Chest* **90** 243–246

Baumgartner JE, Rachlin JR, Beckstead JH *et al* (1990) Primary central nervous system lymphomas: natural history and response to radiation therapy in patients with acquired immunodeficiency syndrome. *Journal of Neurosurgery* **73** 206–211

Beral V, Peterman TA, Berkelman RL and Jaffe HW (1990) Kaposi's sarcoma among persons with AIDS: a sexually transmitted infection? *Lancet* **i** 123–128

Bermudez MA, Grant KM, Rodvien R and Mendes F (1989) Non-Hodgkin's lymphoma in a population with or at risk for acquired immunodeficiency syndrome: indications for intensive chemotherapy. *American Journal of Medicine* **86** 71–76.

Burkes RL, Meyer PL, Gill PS, Parker JL, Rasheed S and Levine A (1986) Rectal lymphoma in homosexual men. *Archives of Internal Medicine* **146** 913–915

Centers for Disease Control (1982) Diffuse undifferentiated non-Hodgkin's lymphoma among homosexual males—United States. *Morbidity Mortality Weekly Report* **31** 277–279

Centers for Disease Control (1985) Revision of the case definition of acquired immunodeficiency syndrome for national reporting: United States. *Morbidity Mortality Weekly Report* **31** 373–375

Centers for Disease Control (1990) *HIV/AIDS Surveillance Report*, pp 1–22. Centers for Disease Control, Atlanta, Georgia

Ciricillo SF and Rosenblum ML (1990) Use of CT and MR imaging to distinguish intracranial lesions and to define the need for biopsy in AIDS patients. *Journal of Neurosurgery* **73**

720–724

Connors JM and Klimo P (1988) Chemotherapy for malignant lymphomas and related conditions: 1987 update and additional observations. *Seminars in Hematology* **25 (Supplement 2)** 41–46

DeVita VT, Hubbard SM, Young RC and Longo DL (1988) The role of chemotherapy in diffuse aggressive lymphomas. *Seminars in Hematology* **25 (Supplement 2)** 2–10

Formenti SC, Gill PS, Lean E, Rarick M, Meyer PR, Boswell W, Petrovich Z, Chak L and Levine AM (1989) Primary central nervous system lymphoma in AIDS: Results of radiation therapy. *Cancer* **63** 1101–1107

Freter CE (1990) Acquired immunodeficiency syndrome-associated lymphomas. *Journal of the National Cancer Institute (USA) Monograph* **10** 45–54

Friedman SL (1988) Gastrointestinal and hepatobiliary neoplasms in AIDS. *Gastroenterology Clinics of North America* **17** 465–486

Gill PS, Levine AM, Krailo M *et al* (1987) AIDS-related malignant lymphoma: results of prospective treatment trials. *Journal of Clinical Oncology* **5** 1322–1328

Gill PS, Levine AM, Meyer PR *et al* (1985) Primary central nervous system lymphoma in homosexual men: clinical, immunologic, and pathologic features. *American Journal of Medicine* **78** 742–748

Guarner J, Brynes RK, Chan WC, Birdsong G and Hertxler G (1987) Primary non-Hodgkin's lymphoma of the heart in two patients with the acquired immunodeficiency syndrome. *Archives of Pathology and Laboratory Medicine* **111** 254–256

Hanto DW, Frizzera G, Gajl-Peczalkska K *et al* (1981) Clinical spectrum of lymphoproliferative disorders in renal transplant recipients and evidence for the role of Epstein-Barr virus. *Cancer Research* **41** 4253–4266

Holland HK, Saral R, Rossi JJ *et al* (1989) Allogeneic bone marrow transplantation, zidovudine, and human immunodeficiency virus type (HIV-1) infection: studies in a patient with non-Hodgkin's lymphoma. *Annals of Internal Medicine* **11** 973–981

Italian Cooperative Group for AIDS-related Tumours (1988) Malignant lymphomas in patients with or at risk for AIDS in Italy. *Journal of the National Cancer Institute (USA)* **80** 855–860

Kalter SP, Riggs SA, Cabanillas F *et al* (1985) Aggressive non-Hodgkin's lymphomas in immunocompromised homosexual males. *Blood* **66** 655–659

Kaplan LD, Abrams DI, Feigal E *et al* (1989a) AIDS-associated non-Hodgkin's lymphoma in San Francisco. *Journal of the American Medical Association* **261** 719–724

Kaplan LD, Kahn J, Jacobson M, Bottles K and Cello J (1989b) Primary bile duct lymphoma in the acquired immunodeficiency syndrome. *Annals of Internal Medicine* **110** 161–162

Kaplan LD, Kahn JO, Crowe S *et al* (1991) Clinical and virologic effects of recombinant human granulocyte-macrophage colony-stimulating factor (rGM-CSF) in patients receiving chemotherapy for HIV-associated non-Hodgkin's lymphoma: results of a randomized trial. *Journal of Clinical Oncology* (in press)

Knowles DM, Chamulak GA, Subar M *et al* (1988) Lymphoid neoplasia associated with the acquired immunodeficiency syndrome (AIDS). *Annals of Internal Medicine* **108** 744–753

Levine AM, Wernz JC, Kaplan L *et al* (1989) Low dose chemotherapy with CNS prophylaxis and zidovudine (AZT) maintenance for AIDS-related lymphoma: follow up data from a multi-institutional trial. *Blood* **74 (Supplement 1)** 239a

Levine AS, Gill PS, Meyer PR *et al* (1985) Retrovirus and malignant lymphoma in homosexual men. *Journal of the American Medical Association* **254** 1921–1925

Lowenthal DA, Straus DJ, Campbell SW, Gold JWM, Clarkson BD and Koziner B (1988) AIDS-related lymphoid neoplasia: The Memorial Hospital experience. *Cancer* **61** 2325–2337

Navia BA, Petito CK, Gold JW, Cho E, Jordan BD and Price RW (1986) Cerebral toxoplasmosis complicating the acquired immune deficiency syndrome: clinical and neuropathological findings in patients. *Annals of Neurology* **19** 224–238

Nyberg DA, Jeffrey RB, Federle MP, Bottles K and Abrams DI (1986) AIDS-related lymphomas: evaluation by abdominal CT. *Radiology* **159** 59–63

Penn I (1983) Lymphomas complicating organ transplantation. *Transplantation Proceedings* **15 (Supplement 1)** 2790–2797

Pluda JM, Yarchoan R, Jaffe ES *et al* (1990) Development of non-Hodgkin lymphoma in a cohort of patients with severe human immunodeficiency virus (HIV) infection on long-term antiretroviral therapy. *Annals of Internal Medicine* **113** 276–282

Polish LB, Cohn DL, Ryder JW, Myers AM and O'Orien RF (1989) Pulmonary non-Hodgkin's lymphoma in AIDS. *Chest* **96** 1321–1326

Purtilo DT (1980) Epstein-Barr virus-induced oncogenesis in immune-deficient individuals. *Lancet* **i** 300–303

Remick SC, Diamond C, Migliozzi JA *et al* (1990) Primary central nervous system lymphoma in patients with and without the acquired immune deficiency syndrome. *Medicine (Baltimore)* **69** 345–360

So YT, Beckstead JH and Davis RL (1986) Primary central nervous system lymphoma in acquired immune deficiency syndrome: a clinical and pathologic study. *Annals of Neurology* **20** 566–572

Ziegler JL, Drew WL, Miner RC *et al* (1982) Outbreak of Burkitt's-like lymphoma in homosexual men. *Lancet* **ii** 631–633

Ziegler JL, Beckstead JA, Volberding PA *et al* (1984) Non-Hodgkin's lymphoma in homosexual men: relation to generalized lymphadenopathy and the acquired immunodeficiency syndrome. *New England Journal of Medicine* **311** 565–570

The authors are responsible for the accuracy of the references.

Surgical Pathology of HIV Associated Lymphoproliferations

B G HERNDIER

Departments of Pathology and Laboratory Medicine, University of California San Francisco, San Francisco General Hospital, San Francisco, California 94110

INTRODUCTION: HISTOLOGY

Since near the beginning of the perceived AIDS epidemic, it has been clear that patients with HIV disease manifest a variety of lymphoproliferations of concern to the surgical pathologist. The lesions range from the devastating lymphoma (non-Hodgkin lymphoma) (Ziegler *et al*, 1984; Levine, 1987), to the often indolent persistent generalized lymphadenopathy (Meyer *et al*, 1984; Abrams, 1986) associated with the AIDS related complex to the HIV Epstein-Barr virus (EBV) lymphoproliferations of children such as lymphocytic interstitial pneumonitis (Liebow and Carrington, 1973; Kradin *et al*, 1982; Rubenstein, 1986). Diagnostic accuracy is critical, since the managements of lymphoma, Hodgkin's disease and persistent generalized lymphadenopathy are radically different and constantly evolving as clinicians tackle the problems associated with the use of cytotoxic therapies in the setting of immunodeficiency. Therapy is further complicated by concomitant anti-HIV therapies and management of often simultaneous opportunistic infections. The following chapter is not an exhaustive survey of lymphoproliferations in HIV disease but reflects current diagnostic concerns encountered at San Francisco General Hospital (SFGH), a public hospital with a high HIV prevalence and employing innovative protocols addressing various facets of HIV disease. This chapter will not discuss in detail fundamental haematolymphoid pathology. There are many monographs available that give excellent descriptions and definitions of "lymphoma", Hodgkin's disease, follicular hyperplasia of lymph nodes etc (Dorfman and Warnke, 1974; Jaffe, 1985).

Histological Subtypes of HIV Lymphoma

The classification used at SFGH (the Working Formulation) differs from the usual classification of lymphomas (reviewed by Burke, 1990) and was based on an attempt to relate the morphological subtypes to the ultimate prognosis. The vast majority of HIV lymphomas, approximately 90%, "fit" into three histological subtypes according to the Working Formulation (Dorfman et al, 1982): small non-cleaved cell lymphoma (SNC), large cell immunoblastic lymphoma (IBL) and large cell lymphoma (LCL). However, several weaknesses of the Working Formulation become rapidly apparent when faced with the task of accurately classifying HIV lymphomas. One weakness can be roughly traced to the perceived prognostic difference between large cell (intermediate grade) and large cell immunoblastic (high grade) lymphomas used in the Working Formulation cohort. Subsequent studies have not borne out this difference and thus raise the question of the need for this often difficult and subjective histological distinction (Cossman, 1985; Glatstein, 1987). When treating non-HIV lymphomas, an increasing tendency is to use "high grade" curative lymphoma protocols for patients with diffuse lymphomas with significant amounts of large cells whether the large cells are the immunoblasts (central nucleoli) or the so-called lymphoma "large cells" (nucleoli or chromocentres generally apposed to the nuclear membrane). Thus a practical managerial or biologically based classification of non-HIV lymphomas may be evolving from the simple morphological/prognostic classification of the Working Formulation. Clearly, since survival with LCL is not practically different than with the IBL or SNC variety, we tend to perceive and subsequently manage these large cell lymphomas as high grade neoplasms, recognizing the fragile immune system of the host as a major determinant in the ultimate outcome. In our experience, the majority of non-SNC HIV lymphomas tend to show variable mixtures of large cells and immunoblasts (Fig. 1). We tend not to fret about splitting off IBLs from LCLs unless a rare case is clearly composed of a majority of "central nucleoli" immunoblasts. Published monographs, which include photomicrographs from the Working Formulation, leave a great deal of subjective leeway with regard to the IBL/LCL distinction and many HIV cases seem to cluster at this arbitrary dividing line. Thus although we attempt to classify, we recognize the subjective weaknesses of such distinctions.

The classical Burkitt's lymphoma (BL) of children is a distinct histopathological entity. These lymphomas consist of densely packed lymphoblasts interspersed with stainable body macrophages. The individual cells have round hyperchromatic nuclei with small, distinct multiple nucleoli. Wright stained material features intermediate to large blasts with a rim of deeply basophilic

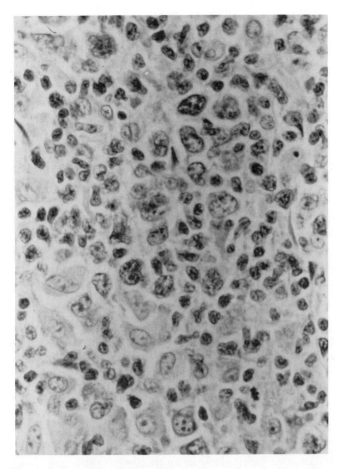

Fig. 1. Large cell lymphoma with a spectrum of atypical lymphocytes admixed with a population of apparently normal macrophages. x270

cytoplasm punctuated by small optically clear vacuoles. Berard and Dorfman (1974) recognized that BL cells derived from adults tended to have greater heterogeneity in cell size than those from children, and thus the designation small non-cleaved non-BL. Studies by Barriga *et al* (1988) and Pelicci *et al* (1986) demonstrated that the endemic as opposed to sporadic (including HIV) forms of BL generally had distinct t(8,14) translocations, the breakpoint being in either the "switch mu" region or the "first intron J_H" region of the immunoglobulin *myc* locus. The above mentioned histological heterogeneity is clearly present in the majority of AIDS associated BL cases, and furthermore, we recognize a subset of cases with the classical BL low power architecture (the so-called starry sky), but the vast majority of the malignant cells are simply quite huge. (We substantiate the "Burkittoid" nature by finding a c-*myc* gene rearrangement pattern by Southern blot analysis of the tumour.) I feel that subclassification should depend on the molecular and immunophenotypic characteristics of each tumour.

Lymphadenopathy in HIV Disease

A large percentage of lymphadenopathies in HIV disease are related to opportunistic infections. The most common occurring at SFGH are mycobacterium avium class (usually diffuse macrophages inspissated with acid fast bacilli, mycobacterium tuberculosis (tends towards a granulomatous presentation), *Cryptococcus neoformans* (unencapsulated forms are often encountered), *Histoplasma capsulatum,* cytomegalovirus and bacterial suppuration. Kaposi's sarcoma (KS) is encountered in lymph nodes and can present diagnostic difficulties, especially with fine needle aspiration biopsies. The foci of KS can be relatively obscure, in a capsular or subcapsular distribution. Kaposi's sarcoma can also be admixed with lymphoma and can be difficult to distinguish from the angioimmunoblastic like lesions often encountered in HIV infected lymph nodes. The consequences of misdiagnosing a subtle KS infected lymph node are not clear, since direct KS therapy is currently reserved for extremely morbid proliferations or cosmetic purposes.

In HIV disease, lymph nodes undergo a variety of temporal changes, probably related to a direct cytopathic effect of the virus and the subsequent immune dysfunction. The patterns of change are summarized in Table 1, which presents significant surgical pathology in HIV lymphadenopathies. This is a highly personalized scheme and actually represents a morphological framework used by our research laboratory (Ng *et al,* 1989; Shiramizu *et al,* 1990; McGrath *et al,* 1991) for studying various aspects of the progression of HIV disease, autoimmune phenomena related to HIV and lymphomagenesis. The hyperplasias (1, 2, 3 in Table 1) are generally present in biopsy specimens from patients early in the course of HIV disease. Lymph node plasmacytosis (4, 5) is a common feature in HIV disease, particularly as an incidental finding in bone marrows and at necropsy. The presence of a major plasma cell infiltrate (we have seen several cases with 30–60% plasma cells) in a bone marrow can at first presentation be quite startling. Ng *et al* (1989) clearly showed that the high incidence of monoclonal and oligoclonal paraproteins in HIV disease is probably due to an attenuated, possibly unregulated, humoral response to HIV. The plasmacytoses are probably the cellular hallmark of the dysfunctional humoral B cell response in HIV disease, which is probably related to CD4+ lymphocyte depletion and the consequent lack of proliferation of CD8+ suppressor cells. A myriad of autoimmune phenomena such as idiopathic thrombocytopaenic purpura, lupus anticoagulants and autoimmune haemolytic anaemia are clinical manifestations of such an inappropriate humoral immune response.

Central Nervous System Lymphoma

Primary central nervous system (CNS) lymphoma is one of the most devastating complications of HIV disease. The average lifespan from diagnosis is of the order of 3 months, significantly shorter than with other initial AIDS diagnoses such as *Pneumocystis carinii* pneumonia and even the peripheral lymphomas

TABLE 1. Patterns of lymphadenopathy in HIV disease

Pattern	Comments
(1) Follicular hyperplasia	Early response to HIV
(2) Follicular hyperplasia with cytopathological signs	Fusion of monocytes/CD4$^+$ cells (HIV mediated), focal lymphocyte depletion (germinal centres), early loss of dendritic reticular pattern
(3) Diffuse reactive hyperplasia	Mixed B, T cells, minimal lymphoid atypia, loss of follicular architecture
(4) Angioimmunoblastic like lesions	Increased vascularity, no follicular architecture, mixed T, B cells, macrophages (often HIV infected) +/– atypical large cells/immunoblasts +/– plasmacytosis, proteinaceous deposits
(5) Lymphoid depletion	Node framework vascularity prominent +/– atypical lymphocytes/R-S cells +/– plasmacytosis
(6) Frank diffuse lymphoma	Defined as having a dominant component of large cells/immunoblasts in a diffuse infiltrative pattern
(7) Frank Hodgkin's disease	Presence of R-S cells and variants thereof, reactive background such as (3) (4) (5) above (background lymphocytes often are atypical in HIV Hodgkin's disease, leuM1 type markers can be useful in this setting but can be positive in the setting of cytomegalovirus inflammations and other reactive conditions)

(non-CNS lymphomas). Although BL cytology is encountered, the majority of the CNS lymphomas are of the large cell and/or immunoblastic types. Tumour necrosis and distinct vasocentric growth patterns are often prominent.

Our extensive clinical experience at SFGH suggests that early diagnosis and subsequent clinical management of CNS lymphomas, in particular with radiotherapy, will lead to improved survival (Baumgartner *et al,* 1990). For early diagnosis, the role of the surgical pathologist is central and difficult. The criteria for CNS lymphoma and for cerebral toxoplasmosis are for the most part formed from impressions gathered on necropsy material or from biopsy specimens garnered from full blown disease states. Diagnostic difficulty arises because these criteria are often irrelevant in the setting of the frozen section, the minute brain biopsy and early disease (Fig. 2).

At SFGH, the HIV infected patient or patient "at risk for AIDS" with a radiologically defined CNS mass (usually via CT or MR scan; Ciricillo and Rosenblum 1990) is serologically tested for toxoplasmosis. Positive toxoserology is usually followed by a short closely monitored trial of anti-toxoplasma medication. Brain biopsy is required if there is no significant radiological or clinical improvement. Negative toxoserology necessitates an immediate brain biopsy. The surgical pathologist's usual first role is to assist the surgeon in the accurate localization of the CNS lesion by frozen section interpretation. The

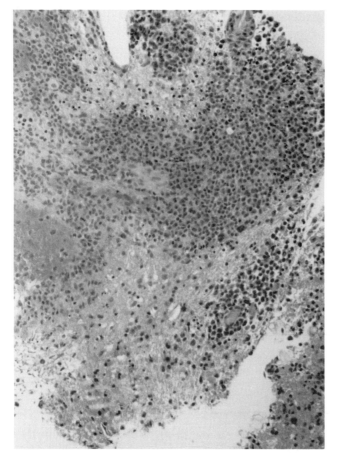

Fig. 2. Diagnostic fragment of CNS lymphoma. x135

intraoperative goal should be minimal—to determine whether sufficient tissue has been procured for later final diagnosis on permanent section. Necrotic foci (as opposed to lymphoma tumour necrosis), gliosis and aggregates of granulocytes usually indicate toxoplasmosis. Occasionally, a diagnostic toxo-pseudocyst can be seen on frozen section. Although aggregates of lymphocytes can be present in toxoplasmosis, these are mostly associated with lymphoma, particularly if the lymphocytes are atypical, in a perivascular distribution or in great numbers. The presence of bizarre astrocytes, darkly staining large oligodendroglial cells and minimum inflammation indicate progressive multi-focal leukodystrophy (PML). Under no circumstances should the pathologist or surgeon be satisfied with the frozen section diagnosis of simply "gliosis"—subsequent permanent sections can be non-diagnostic. Pan cultures of biopsy specimens are in order if there is any suspicion of an infectious aetiology.

On permanent sections, the three major CNS diagnoses in AIDS are lymphoma, toxoplasmosis and PML. An excellent monograph describing the basic pathology of these lesions and the diffuse CNS pathology of HIV disease is that by Sotrel (1989). Baumgartner *et al* (1990) reported the CNS lymphomas to be monoclonal EBV associated B cell proliferations. However, we have subsequently encountered diagnostic CNS lymphoma biopsies that featured immunophenotypic mixtures of B and T lymphocytes or polyclonal B cell proliferations by Southern blot analysis of immunoglobulin gene rearrangements. Clearly, larger series of clinical data on CNS lymphoma emphasizing histological, immunodiagnostic and molecular correlations are required to evaluate the utility of special studies in difficult surgical pathology cases.

Surgical Pathology Problems in Staging HIV Lymphoma

Initial staging of HIV lymphoma at SFGH necessitates a staging bone marrow biopsy. Approximately 30% of the patients will have bone marrow involvement (Kaplan *et al*, 1989). In general, lymphomatous involvement of the bone marrow is obvious. However, a few cases have shown small clusters of, or single, atypical lymphocytes. The distinction between early marrow involvement with lymphoma and the common background lymphoplasmacytoses in HIV infected marrows can be difficult to see.

In our experience (Northfelt *et al*, 1990), the establishment of the initial diagnosis of lymphoma by a bone marrow biopsy during cytopaenia/fever workup is rare (0/50 in a 2 year span). Northfelt *et al* (1990) further discuss the controversial role of the bone marrow in ruling out disseminated fungal/mycobacterium infections in the HIV infected patient.

The surgical pathologist and cytologist in busy AIDS hospitals are often confronted with difficult decisions regarding malignant effusions (pleural, ascitic and to a lesser extent the cerebrospinal fluid). Early in the AIDS epidemic, several cases of "malignant" lymphoid effusions were diagnosed on the basis of monomorphous suspensions of apparent "immunoblasts" or large lymphoid cells. However, clinical follow-up of some cases designated as "malignant" effusions cast doubt on the appropriateness of these diagnoses. Spontaneous clinical resolution of the effusion could occur, and in some cases examined at necropsy, there were insignificant effusions and no evidence of a lymphomatous mass lesion. As we became more aware of polyclonal lymphomas in tissue (see below), it followed that "malignant" appearing polyclonal lymphoproliferations could be a component of effusions in HIV infected patients. The net result of these observations is an avoidance of diagnosing malignancies in fluids from HIV infected patients; instead, we use such terms as "atypical lymphocytosis" and suggest close clinical observation. On occasion, very anaplastic lymphoid cells or cells with characteristic BL morphology are encountered, and we have subsequently made a diagnosis of lymphoma (subsequent gene rearrangement studies did indeed show a monoclonal B cell process). Overall, we feel that criteria for judging malignant effusions in HIV disease are ill defined and require a much larger body of clinicopathological correlation.

UTILITY OF IMMUNOPHENOTYPIC AND MOLECULAR ANALYSIS IN THE DIAGNOSIS OF HIV ASSOCIATED LYMPHOPROLIFERATIONS

Immunohistochemistry

The mainstay of the diagnosis of lymphoma in the setting of HIV disease is histological evaluation. In our opinion, although others differ, immunohisto-chemistry is of marginal value in separating benign from malignant conditions in HIV disease and can actually be misleading. Two basic rules for using im-munohistochemistry as an adjunct to histology in formulating a diagnosis will be discussed.

a. A "monoclonal" lymphoproliferation does not necessarily imply malignancy.
b. Polyclonal lymphoproliferations are not necessarily benign.

The example of plasmacytoses in HIV disease has been discussed above—the apparent monoclonal and oligoclonal paraproteins are probably a result of at-tenuated immune responses to HIV or dysfunctional regulation of the humoral immune response. A more serious error is the false light chain restriction study. Basically, this is a result of failure of either the primary kappa or lambda reagents, giving an impression of monoclonality. Unfortunately, positive con-trol tissue can create a false sense of security, since the failure of the light chain reagents is often dependent on the diagnostic tissue. This type of error is not unique to HIV infected tissue.

A more common diagnostic misinterpretation made with biopsy specimens from HIV infected patients is the false positive polyclonal proliferation. We commonly encounter combination strong kappa and lambda staining on paraf-fin, plastic or frozen sections. Using a cytofluorograph, this non-specific pat-tern can be traced to individual B cells binding both the kappa and lambda pri-mary antibody reagents. The phenomenon is probably a function of the patient's hypergammaglobulinaemia, with an autoimmune component reacting in a "rheumatoid factor" manner to cell surface immunoglobulins. Therefore, we tend not to use light chain exclusion via immunostaining for clinical deci-sion making in HIV disease and prefer molecular biological determinations of clonality (limitations of these techniques are discussed below). However, it should be noted that other laboratories have published immunohistochemical light chain studies on HIV lymphomas and may indeed use the technique in clinical settings (Meyer *et al*, 1985).

Two other immunohistochemical approaches based on the following as-sumptions are theoretically possible for delineation of benign and malignant lymphoproliferations.

a. Diffuse reactive hyperplasias tend to be mixtures of B and T cells.
b. Lymphomas have abnormal immunophenotypes (Uckun, 1990).

In non-HIV lymphomas, the concept of the T cell rich monoclonal B cell lymphoma is becoming established in the literature (Picker *et al*, 1987). We find a similar phenomenon in HIV disease with two key differences: (1) the T cells (up to 70% in some cases) generally appear as "activated" large cells, not as an infiltrate of small lymphocytes; (2) the B cell proliferation is polyclonal in nature (by Southern blot analysis). Thus the proliferation appears to be a monomorphous population of large cells and immunoblasts, ie a histologically defined lymphoma. Despite the immunophenotypic impression of a reactive mixture, these proliferations are not benign processes. We bolster this impression of malignancy by using such simple criteria as widespread organ destruction (lung, liver and heart are common sites) and inferring the lymphoproliferation as causing significant morbidity and early death in the context of HIV disease.

Do B cells in HIV lymphomas have unusual diagnostically useful phenotypes? The lymphoma B cells express surface IgM, CD20 (leu26), with variable expression of CD19, CD22. Rare cases, usually BL, exhibit cALLa positivity (CD10). CD5 (leu1) is rarely expressed. Unusual is the universal lack of expression of CD21 and, in a limited survey (six lymphomas to date), CD23. This phenotype has important ramifications in the pathogenesis of HIV lymphomas. CD21, or the CR2 complement receptor, is the initial attachment receptor of EBV (Fingeroth *et al*, 1984). CD23 is the low affinity IgE receptor upregulated by either interleukin-4 (a T cell derived glycoprotein [Galizzi *et al*, 1988]) or EBV B cell infection. The upregulation of CD23 is a result of the EBNA-2 gene product, as indicated by the differential transfection studies of Wang *et al* (1987). The lack of CD21, CD23 antigens and the relative paucity of molecular evidence of EBV in the non-CNS lymphomas (see molecular biology discussion below) would on first approximation minimize the role of EBV in HIV associated lymphomagenesis. Diagnostically, this unusual lymphoma phenotype is useless, for we also find diffuse reactive hyperplasias in HIV infected nodes also feature B cells lacking in CD21, CD23 antigens. Early follicular hyperplasia in HIV disease features clustering of CD21, CD23 positive cells in germinal centres. This apparent temporal disappearance of CD21 and CD23 B cells in HIV disease could be due to an elimination of viral antigen expression in EBV infected cells (Birx *et al*, 1986) during the course of the disease. However, such mechanisms are currently speculative.

Molecular Biology of HIV Associated Lymphoproliferations

In our experience, the peripheral lymphomas associated with HIV infection can be roughly divided into two categories: (1) a monoclonal proliferation with either rearrangement of the c-*myc* proto-oncogene or clonal infection with EBV; (2) a polyclonal proliferation of B cells, by definition lacking a clonal c-*myc* rearrangement and often lacking EBV genomes (Fig. 3). In a molecular analysis of 39 lymphomas, almost 44% fit into the latter interesting category (Shiramizu *et al*, 1990). Generally, the polyclonal lymphomas are of LCL/IBL histology and are often composed of mixtures of "activated" appearing B and T cells.

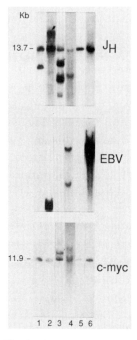

Fig. 3. Southern blot molecular phenotypes of HIV lymphomas, the SFGH experience. J_H restriction enzymes are *Hind*III plus *Eco*R1 (Ravetch *et al*, 1981), EBV restriction enzymes are *Bam*H1, the probe is from the terminal repeat (Raab-Traub and Flynn, 1986), c-*myc* restriction enzyme is *Eco*R1 and the probe is from the 3rd exon (Dalla-Favera *et al*, 1983). Lanes 5 and 6 represent polyclonal lymphomas. Lanes 1–4 represent molecular phenotypes of monoclonal tumours

The existence of polyclonal "lymphomas" is a controversial issue in HIV disease (Knowles *et al*, 1988); however, they have been described in some reports in AIDS (Levine, 1987; Lippman *et al*, 1988). Despite this controversy, the concept of the polyclonal lymphoma in the iatrogenically immunosuppressed transplant patient is well established (Frizzera *et al*, 1981; Hanto *et al*, 1983; Starzl *et al*, 1984). The lymphoproliferations in the congenital immunodeficiencies (Purtilo, 1981; Penn, 1986) are associated with EBV, similar to the transplant lymphomas. As in the transplant and immunodeficiency lymphomas described by Frizzera *et al* (1980, 1981), we note a high incidence of extranodal presentation, a "geographic" tumour necrosis and an often polymorphous appearance—admixtures of immunoblasts, large cells, "plasmacytoid cells," occasional small lymphocytes and even macrophages (Fig. 1).

Since the concept of the polyclonal lymphomas in HIV disease is somewhat controversial and depends to a large extent on definition, I will attempt to convey our definition of the histological and molecular parameters of high grade lymphomas in HIV disease. Indicators of malignancy are progressive extensive tissue destruction and rapidly fatal natural course of disease. In a necropsy series of polyclonal B cell lymphomas, analyzed at multiple tumour sites, we demonstrated widespread organ involvement and were reasonably certain the tumours were important in accelerating the patients' deaths (McGrath *et al*, 1991). The histology of these lesions fit traditional surgical pathology definitions of lymphoma (Dorfman RF, personal communication)— proliferations of large cells/immunoblasts often mixed with patches of tumour necrosis. Sites designated polyclonal by immunoglobulin gene rearrangement studies were histologically identical to monoclonal sites in the same patient. With the knowledge gained from the necropsies, we felt confident that our diagnoses of surgical biopsies were not in error—the biopsies did not represent mere diffuse polyclonal hyperplasias but bona fide lymphomas deserving of oncological intervention.

Fastidious attention to handling of tissue specimens is required to define a tumour as polyclonal by gene rearrangement studies. Each biopsy specimen is divided, tissue is submitted for classical surgical pathology evaluation and adjacent sections are frozen at $-70^\circ C$ for later DNA extraction. No cell lines allowed! Cell lines are inevitably monoclonal. At DNA extraction, reverification of histology and an immunophenotype is performed on the frozen section. DNA extraction, restriction digests, electrophoresis and probing (J_H probes for the immunoglobulin locus, $C_T\beta$ for the T cell antigen receptor locus) were slight variations of the initial descriptions of Korsmeyer *et al* (1983) and Cossman *et al* (1988). We defined a clonal population as the emergence of a band at 5% of the genomic DNA. Standard DNA was extracted from a germline source such as the liver and "spiked" with a rearranged band at 5% the concentration of the germline source. The DNA for the 5% "spike" was extracted from known monoclonal B cell or T cell lines. The use of an internal standard on a given electrophoretic run prevents misinterpretation of overexposed gels. Insignificant Southern blot bands from reactive lymphoid clones or small subsets of tumour should not be construed as being representative of the whole tumour. These types of misinterpretation are examples of "false positive" diagnoses of a monoclonal process. Remember, even at our definition of 5% DNA in a rearranged band, at least 20, probably more, clones of B cells or T cells are potentially present in the tumour.

Unfortunately for the surgical pathologist, the existence of polyclonal lymphomas in HIV disease renders molecular biology relatively impotent in making the distinction between benign and malignant conditions. Monoclonal lymphomas usually present little histological challenge, and many fall into the BL histological category. For HIV biopsies, we virtually never request gene rearrangement studies (although others consider this of value) to help diagnose a histologically ambiguous case—a Southern blot interpretation of "polyclonal" could represent either a polyclonal lymphoma or a lymphoid hyperplasia. Currently, we are developing clinical protocols examining stratification of lymphomas into polyclonal or monoclonal designations (see Northfelt and Kaplan, this issue). The working hypothesis is that polyclonal lymphomas will show some degree of reversibility with immunomodulatory or "immunosparing" therapies, analogous to the transplant lymphomas.

Similarly, determination of clonality by Southern blot analysis of circularized terminal repeats of the EBV (Cleary *et al*, 1988) and c-*myc* rear-rangements (Shiramizu *et al*, 1990) suffers from the above interpretative limitations of clonality determination by immunoglobulin or T cell antigen receptor gene rearrangements. Furthermore, we find that only a fraction of the AIDS lymphomas are associated with EBV at the 1% detection sensitivity (36%) or have detectable c-*myc* rearrangements (23%) (Shiramizu *et al*, 1990).

CONCLUSION

The surgical pathologist should be familiar with the variety of histological profiles of the lymphoproliferations in HIV disease. Proliferative states such as follicular hyperplasias and granulomata reflect immunological reactivity to HIV and the myriad of opportunistic infections. HIV dependent degradation of the immune system is histologically represented by the atypical hyperplasias such as the angioimmunoblastic like lesions, plasmacytoses and lymphoid depleted states. The most important lymphoproliferative lesions from a managerial standpoint are the lymphomas and Hodgkin's disease. Histological evaluation is the mainstay of diagnosis. Moreover, immunophenotypic and molecular clonality studies to augment histological impressions can be easily misinterpreted if one is not aware of the existence of polyclonal lymphomas in AIDS. Central nervous system lymphomas present diagnostic challenges by virtue of the small biopsy sizes and the need for accurate frozen section interpretation during surgery.

The diagnosis of Hodgkin's disease depends on the coexistence of Reed-Sternberg cells and variants thereof in a mixed inflammatory background. Levine (1987) noted the clinical parallels between Hodgkin's disease and the high grade lymphomas in HIV disease. Hodgkin's disease in HIV infected patients often presents in advanced stages, appears to be clinically aggressive and frequently occupies extranodal sites. The mixed inflammatory background of Hodgkin's disease is by virtual definition a polyclonal proliferation of B and T cells. We and other surgical pathologists have noted the frequent atypical nature of lymphoid cells in the HIV associated Hodgkin's disease background and occasional cases with a paucity of Reed-Sternberg variants. The diagnosis of Hodgkin's disease in some difficult cases was to a large extent made on the basis of leuM1 immunostaining, but it should be noted that the specificity of this reagent and other "Reed-Sternberg" antibodies has always been questionable, especially in light of recent reports of crossreactivity to cytomegalovirus (Rushin *et al*, 1990). These atypical mixed B and T cell Hodgkin's disease backgrounds are somewhat similar to a subset of HIV lymphomas we have analyzed that feature phenotypic mixtures of lymphocytes which are polyclonal by gene rearrangement studies. Furthermore, our polyclonal HIV lymphomas are mostly EBV negative (14/17), a frequency not unlike that reported by Weiss *et al* (1989) for non-HIV Hodgkin's disease (13/16). The pathogenetic significance of this lack of EBV involvement in the polyclonal HIV lymphomas and Hodgkin's disease is unclear. We are nevertheless intrigued by similarities between these two neoplasms and hypothesize that they exist on a diagnostic, pathogenetic and even aetiological continuum.

Diagnostic problems and controversies exist with regard to characterizing HIV associated lymphoproliferations. Building on the present base of knowledge, we plan to continue to refine diagnostic acumen and to resolve clinically important controversies with further correlative studies.

SUMMARY

The surgical pathologist is confronted with a variety of lymphoproliferative states in the setting of HIV disease. Classifying lymphomas, differentiating benign and malignant disease, accurate staging and identifying non-neoplastic lymphadenopathies still rely on histological evaluation as the mainstay of diagnosis. Immunophenotypic and molecular analysis have offered considerable insight into the pathology of HIV associated lymphoproliferations but must be used with caution as diagnostic tools in HIV disease.

References

Abrams DI (1986) Lymphadenopathy related to the AIDS in homosexual men. *Medical Clinics of North America* **70** 693–706

Barriga F, Kiwanuka J, Alvarez-Mon M *et al* (1988) Significance of chromosome 8 breakpoint location in Burkitt's lymphoma: correlation with geographical origin and association with Epstein-Barr virus. *Current Topics in Microbiology and Immunology* **141** 128–136

Baumgartner JE, Rachlin JR, Beckstead JH *et al* (1990) Primary central nervous system lymphomas: natural history and response to radiation therapy in 55 patients with acquired immunodeficiency syndrome. *Journal of Neurosurgery* **73** 206–211

Berard CW and Dorfman RF (1974) Histopathology of malignant lymphomas. *Clinical Hematology* **3** 39–76

Birx DL, Redfield RR and Tosato G (1986) Defective regulation of Epstein-Barr virus infection in patients with acquired immunodeficiency syndrome (AIDS) or AIDS-related disorders. *New England Journal of Medicine* **314** 874–879

Burke JS (1990) The histopathologic classifiation of non-Hodgkin's lymphomas: ambiguities in the working formulation and two newly reported categories. *Seminars in Oncology* **Vol 17** 3–10

Ciricillo SF and Rosenblum ML (1990) Use of CT and MR imaging to distinguish intracranial lesions and to define the need for biopsy in AIDS patients. *Journal of Neurosurgery* **73** 720–724

Cleary ML, Nalesnik MA, Shearer WT and Sklar J (1988) Clonal analysis of transplant-associated lymphoproliferations based on the structure of the genomic termini of the Epstein-Barr virus. *Blood* **72** 349–352

Cossman J (1985) Diffuse, agressive non-Hodgkin's lymphomas, In: Jaffe ES (ed). *Surgical Pathology of the Lymph Nodes and Related Organs*, pp 203–217, WB Saunders, Philadelphia

Cossman J, Uppenkamp M, Sundeen J, Coupland R and Raffeld M (1988) Molecular genetics and the diagnosis of lymphoma. *Archives of Pathology and Laboratory Medicine* **112** 117–127

Crowe S, Mills J and McGrath MS (1987) Quantitative immunocytofluorographic analysis of

CD4 surface antigen expression and HIV infection of human peripheral blood monocyte/macrophages. *AIDS Research and Human Retroviruses* **3** 135–145

Dalla-Favera R, Matinotti S, Gallo RC, Erickson J and Croce CM (1983) Translocation and rearrangements of the c-myc oncogene locus in human undifferentiated B cell lymphomas. *Science* **219** 963–967

Dorfman RF, Burke JS and Berard CW (1982) A working formulation of non-Hodgkin's lymphomas: background, recommendations, histological criteria, and relationship to other classifications, In: Rosenberg S and Kaplan HS (eds). *Malignant Lymphomas*, pp 351–368, Academic Press, Inc, New York

Dorfman RF and Warnke R (1974) Lymphadenopathy stimulating the malignant lymphomas. *Human Pathology* **5** 519–550

Fingeroth JD, Weis JJ, Tedder TF, Strominger JL, Biro PA and Fearon DT (1984) Epstein-Barr virus receptor of human B lymphocytes is the C3d receptor CR2. *Proceedings of the National Academy of Sciences of the USA* **81** 4510–4514

Frizzera G, Rosai J, Dehner LP, Spector BD and Kersey JH (1980) Lymphoreticular disorders in primary immunodeficiencies: new findings based on an up-to-date histologic classification of 35 cases. *Cancer* **46** 692–699

Frizzera G, Hanto DW, Gajl-Peczalska KJ *et al* (1981) Polymorphic diffuse B cell hyperplasias and lymphomas in renal transplant recipients. *Cancer Research* **41** 4262–4279

Galizzi J-P, Cabrillat H, Rousset F, Menetrier C, deVries JE and Banchereau J (1988) IFN- and prostaglandin E2 inhibit IL-4-induced expression of Fc R2/CD23 on B lymphocytes through different mechanisms without altering binding of IL-4 to its receptor. *Journal of Immunology* **141** 1982–1988

Glatstein E (1987) Lymphomania: non-Hodgkin's lymphoma as possibly viewed through the eyes of Lewis Carroll. *Journal of the Royal Society of Medicine* **80** 71–75

Hanto DW, Gail-Peczalska KJ, Frizzera G *et al* (1983) Epstein-Barr virus (EBV) induced polyclonal and monoclonal B cell lymphoproliferative diseases occurring after renal transplantation. Clinical, pathologic, and virologic findings and implications for therapy. *Annals of Surgery* **198** 356–368

Jaffe ES (ed) (1985) *Surgical Pathology of the Lymph Nodes and Related Organs*. WB Saunders, Philadelphia

Kaplan CD, Abrams D, Feigal E *et al* (1989) AIDS associated non-Hodgkin's lymphoma in San Francisco. *Journal of the American Medical Association* **261** 719–724

Knowles DM, Chamulak GA, Subar M *et al* (1988) Lymphoid neoplasia associated with the acquired immunodeficiency syndrome (AIDS). *Annals of Internal Medicine* **108** 744–753

Korsmeyer SJ, Arnold A, Bakshi A *et al* (1983) Immunoglobulin gene rearrangement and cell surface antigen expression in acute lymphocytic leukemias of T cell and B cell precursor origins. *Journal of Clinical Investigation* **71** 301–31

Kradin RL, Young RH, Kradin L and Mark E (1982) Immunoblastic lymphoma arising in chronic lymphoid hyperplasia of the pulmonary interstitium. *Cancer* **50** 1339–1343

Levine AM (1987) Non-Hodgkin's lymphomas and other malignancies in AIDS. *Seminars in Oncology* **14** 34–39

Liebow AA and Carrington CB (1973) Diffuse pulmonary lymphoreticular infiltration associated with dysproteinemia. *Medical Clinics of North America* **57** 809–843

Lippman SM, Volk JR, Spier CM and Grogan TM (1988) Clonal ambiguity of human immunodeficiency virus-associated lymphomas. *Archives of Pathology and Laboratory Medicine* **112** 128–132

McGrath MS, Hwang KM, Caldwell SE *et al* (1989) GLQ223: an inhibitor of human immunodeficiency virus replication in acutely and chronically infected cells of lymphocyte and mononuclear phagocyte lineage. *Proceedings of the National Academy of Sciences of the USA* **86** 2844–3848

McGrath MS, Shiramizu B, Meeker T, Kaplan L and Herndier B (1991) AIDS-associated polyclonal lymphoma: identification of a new HIV-associated disease process. *Journal of*

Acquired Immune Deficiency Syndrome 4 408–415

Meyer PR, Yanagihara ET, Parker JW and Lukes RJ (1984) A distinctive follicular hyperplasia in the acquired immunodeficiency syndrome (AIDS) and the AIDS related complex. *Hematology Oncology* 2 319–347

Meyer PR, Ormerod LD, Osborn KG *et al* (1985) An immunopathologic evaluation of lymph nodes from monkey and man with acquired immune deficiency syndrome and related conditions. *Hematology Oncology* 3 199–210

Ng V, Chen KH, Hwang KM, Khayam-Bashi H and McGrath MS (1989) The clinical significance of HIV-1 associated paraproteins. *Blood* 74 2471–2475

Northfelt DW, Mayer AJ, Kaplan LD, Abrams DI, Hadley WK and Herndier BG (1990) The utility of bone marrow examination for evaluation of opportunistic infections in patients with HIV-infection. *VI International Conference on AIDS, San Francisco 1990,* Vol 2 p 204

Pelicci P-G, Knowles DM, Arlin ZA *et al* (1986) Multiple monoclonal B cell expansions and c-myc oncogene rearrangement in acquired immune deficiency syndrome-related lymphoproliferative disorders. *Journal of Experimental Medicine* 164 2049–2060

Penn I (1986) The occurrence of malignant tumours in immunosuppressed states, In: Klein E (ed). *Progress in Allergy: AIDS,* Vol 37 pp 259–300, Karger, Basel

Picker LJ, Weiss LM, Medeiros LJ, Wood GS and Warnke RA (1987) Immunophenotypic criteria for the diagnosis of non-Hodgkin's lymphoma. *American Journal of Pathology* 128 181–201

Purtilo DT (1981) Immune deficiency predisposing to Epstein-Barr virus-induced lymphoproliferative diseases: the X-linked lymphoproliferative syndrome as a model. *Advances in Cancer Research* 34 279–312

Raab-Traub N and Flynn K (1986) The structure of the termini of the Epstein-Barr virus as a marker of clonal cellular proliferation. *Cell* 47 883–889

Ravetch JV, Siebenlist U, Korsmeyer S, Waldmann T and Leder P (1981) Structure of the human immunoglobulin mu locus: characterization of embryonic and rearranged J and D genes. *Cell* 27 583–591

Rubinstein A (1986) Pediatric AIDS. In: *Current Problems in Pediatrics,* pp 364–409. Year Book Medical Publishers, Chicago

Rushin JM, Riordan GP, Heaton RB, Sharpe RW, Cotelingam JD and Jaffe ES (1990) Cytomegalovirus-infected cells express leu-M1 antigen: a potential source of diagnostic error. *American Journal of Pathology* 136 989–995

Shiramizu B, Meeker T, Kaplan L, Khayam-Bashi F, Herndier B and McGrath M (1990) Molecular analysis of AIDS-associated lymphoma (AAL). *VI International Conference on AIDS, San Francisco 1990,* Vol 3 p 171

Sotrel A (1989) The nervous system, In: Harawi SJ and O'Hara CJ (eds). *Pathology and Pathophysiology of AIDS and HIV-related Diseases,* pp 201–268, CV Mosby, St Louis

Starzl TE, Nalesnik MA, Porter KA *et al* (1984) Reversibility of lymphomas and lymphoproliferative lesions developing under cyclosporin-steroid therapy. *Lancet* i 583–587

Uckun FM (1990) Regulation of human B cell ontogeny. *Blood* 76 1908–1923

Wang F, Gregory CD, Rowe M *et al* (1987) Epstein-Barr virus nuclear antigen 2 specifically induces expression of the B cell activation antigen CD23. *Proceedings of the National Academy of Sciences of the USA* 84 3452–3456

Weiss LM, Movahed LA, Warnke RA and Sklar J (1989) Detection of Epstein-Barr viral genomes in Reed-Sternberg cells of Hodgkin disease. *New England Journal of Medicine* 320 502–506

Ziegler JL, Beckstead JA, Volberding PA *et al* (1984) Non-Hodgkin's lymphoma in 90 homosexual men: relation to generalized lymphadenopathy and the acquired immunodeficiency syndrome. *New England Journal of Medicine* 311 565–570

The author is responsible for the accuracy of the references.

HIV Infection and Cancers Other Than Non-Hodgkin Lymphoma and Kaposi's Sarcoma

CHARLES S RABKIN • WILLIAM A BLATTNER

Viral Epidemiology Section, National Cancer Institute, Bethesda, Maryland 20892

IMMUNODEFICIENCY AND CANCER

The immune surveillance concept, as formulated by Thomas and extended by Burnet, states that neoplastic cells arise continuously but that they manifest as cancer when cellular immunity fails to control them (Purtilo and Linder, 1983). According to this model, immunosuppression would be expected to have an impact on rates of all types of cancers. However, studies of various populations with immunosuppression, including those with congenital, therapeutic and infectious causes, have identified a much more narrow spectrum of tumour types. Excesses of non-Hodgkin lymphoma and soft tissue sarcomas, especially Kaposi's sarcoma, are particularly prominent in therapeutically immunosuppressed populations and in association with HIV infection. Since non-Hodgkin lymphoma and Kaposi's sarcoma are well recognized outcomes of AIDS, what other tumours might prove to be associated with HIV induced immunosuppression?

Congenital Disorders

The Immunodeficiency Cancer Registry maintained at the University of Minnesota collects case reports of cancers in immunodeficient persons, mainly those with congenitally acquired disorders. The most common malignant disease reported to the Registry is non-Hodgkin lymphoma, accounting for 49%

of the reported cases (Kersey *et al,* 1988); Hodgkin's disease and gastric carcinoma each account for 9% of reported cases (Filipovich *et al,* 1980; Mott 1984). Non-Hodgkin lymphoma occurred in association with a diverse spectrum of immunodeficiency diseases with a broad range of underlying immune defects, including ataxia-telangiectasia, Wiskott-Aldrich syndrome and various immunoglobulin deficiencies. In contrast, gastric carcinomas are primarily reported in patients with common variable immunodeficiency (Filipovich *et al,* 1980). Many of the conditions reported to this registry cause severe immunodeficiency and early death from opportunistic infections, which may limit the associated cancers to those of short latency such as non-Hodgkin lymphoma. Other cancer associations may result from specific defects rather than from immunosuppression per se, for example, ataxia telangectasia-associated myeloid leukaemia, which may be caused by the underlying defect in DNA repair. One limitation of this registry information is that it cannot be used to calculate absolute cancer incidence because the underlying population at risk is uncertain.

Therapeutic Immunosuppression

Another source of information on immunosuppression and cancer are patients whose immune systems have been suppressed by medical treatment. The most striking examples of induced immunosuppression are to be found in transplant recipients. In a Canadian study, transplant patients of Jewish or Mediterranean origin were at 500 times greater risk of Kaposi's sarcoma than controls of similar ancestry, whereas transplant patients of other ancestry were not at increased risk (Harwood *et al,* 1979). The contrast between the striking excess of Kaposi's sarcoma in some HIV infected populations, especially in homosexual men, and a more modest increase in transplant recipients supports the notion that additional factors are important, for example, the postulated occurrence of another sexually acquired agent in homosexual men (Beral *et al,* 1990).

In the USA, kidney transplant recipients proved to have a 35-fold excess risk of non-Hodgkin lymphoma (Hoover and Fraumeni, 1973). The excess was associated with sudden onset of disease and short latency, occurring within the first year after transplantation. The excess risk remained constant for more than 5 years, in parallel with the constant level of immunosuppressive drugs used after transplantation. An excess of squamous cell carcinoma of the skin and lip also occurred, appearing only years after transplantation. Several other cancers were also increased after longer latency, including hepatobiliary carcinoma and soft tissue sarcoma. With longer duration of infection and/or prolonged severe immunodeficiency, HIV infection might also increase the frequency of other tumours.

The collaborative United Kingdom-Australasian study of cancer in patients treated with immunosuppressive drugs found similar excesses of non-Hodgkin lymphoma, squamous cell skin carcinoma and soft tissue sarcoma; cutaneous malignant melanoma was also increased (Kinlen *et al,* 1979). Renal transplant patients and patients receiving immunosuppressive drugs for reasons other than transplantation such as for treatment of severe rheumatoid arthritis proved at increased risk. Thus the excess cancer risk could not be attributable to the transplants themselves.

In a Swedish study, renal transplant recipients were shown to have significant increases in non-Hodgkin lymphoma and squamous cell carcinomas of the lip and perineum, as well as a modest increase in colorectal cancer (Blohme and Brynger, 1985). The relative risks observed in all of these studies are striking, but since transplant patients are under intensive medical follow-up, some of the excess cancers could be an artifact of improved case finding.

HIV AND CANCER

Although only Kaposi's sarcoma and non-Hodgkin lymphoma have been epidemiologically associated with HIV, various other malignant diseases in HIV infected persons have been noted in clinical reports (Robert and Schneiderman, 1984; Kaplan et al, 1987; Ourcy and Jakubek, 1987). On the basis of leads from other disorders of immunity, we and others have attempted to determine whether there are additional HIV related cancers.

Cancer Registry Data

One approach is to examine cancer incidence data obtained from cancer registries. We have examined data from the Surveillance, Epidemiology, and End Results (SEER) Program, which is derived from nine cancer registries covering 10% of the US population. These registries record all incident cancers that occur in residents of their respective areas. Our analyses have focused in particular on single young men in the city of San Francisco, among whom about 20 000 were HIV seropositive in late 1984 (Winkelstein et al, 1987; Bachetti and Moss, 1989).

Analysis of SEER data for 1981–1982 detected a statistically significant increase in the relative incidence of Kaposi's sarcoma and non-Hodgkin lymphoma in these men (Biggar et al, 1985). By 1987, Kaposi's sarcoma had increased 5000-fold and non-Hodgkin lymphoma had increased 10-fold, yet no excess cancers of other tumour types were detected (Table 1; Rabkin et al, 1991). Between 1982 and 1984, hepatocellular carcinoma increased, but this trend did not continue, and the incidence returned to below baseline. Similarly, a small but non-significant increase has lately been noted in anal/anorectal carcinoma. Apart from Kaposi's sarcoma and non-Hodgkin lymphoma, the incidence of all other cancers combined has remained constant. Despite continued surveillance, novel tumour associations have not been demonstrated. Unfortunately, the SEER data do not directly address the question of squamous cell skin carcinoma, since non-melanoma skin cancers are not recorded.

Other investigators have reported that one histological subtype of Hodgkin's disease, mixed cellularity, had increased somewhat in single men

TABLE 1. Relative incidence ratios (taking 1973–1978 rates as a baseline) for selected cancers in single and married men aged 20–49 in San Francisco County, 1979–1987[a]

Tumour	Single				Married			
	1973–78	1979–81	1982–84	1985–87	1973–78	1979–81	1982–84	1985–87
Non-Hodgkin lymphoma	1.0	0.6	2.3	10.4[b]	1.0	1.3	1.2	1.2
Kaposi's sarcoma	1.0	82	2100	5060[b]	1.0	18	14	202[b]
Hodgkin's disease	1.0	0.5	1.3	1.1	1.0	1.0	0.7	1.2
Testicular carcinoma	1.0	1.6	0.9	1.1	1.0	1.3	1.1	1.2
Anal/anorectal carcinoma	1.0	1.7	0.7	2.6	1.0	0	0	0
Hepatocellular carcinoma	1.0	0.3	2.2	0.4	1.0	0.8	1.2	1.2
Oral/pharyngeal/lip carcinoma	1.0	1.2	1.3	1.3	1.0	1.3	0.6	0.6
Melanoma	1.0	0.5	0.7	1.2	1.0	1.0	0.9	0.7

[a]Rabkin et al, 1991
[b]p <0.001 for increasing trend

residing in high AIDS incidence areas of San Francisco (Harnly *et al*, 1989). However, our analyses, with different methods, suggested that the increase was small and did not persist in more recent data.

Analysis of an independent cancer registry in New York detected an increase in anal and anorectal carcinomas which directly preceded the HIV epidemic (Biggar *et al*, 1989). Hodgkin's disease increased abruptly in 1985. Thus an association with HIV infection was uncertain for both of these tumours.

Elem and Patil have examined cancer incidence in Zambia, where there is a substantial epidemic of HIV infection. Apart from Kaposi's sarcoma and non-Hodgkin lymphoma, the total numbers of cancers and their distribution by site have remained constant since 1980 (Elem B and Patil P, personal communication). Cervical cancer data were examined in particular because of a clinical suspicion that the frequency of cervical cancer had increased. Both the total incidence and the age distribution of cases of cervical cancer were stable, suggesting that HIV infection, which occurs in younger individuals, was not a contributing factor (Fig. 1).

The Italian Cooperative Group on AIDS-related Tumors has collected reports of cancer in HIV infected Italians since 1986 (Tirelli *et al*, 1989; Monfardini *et al*, 1990). They have noted that about 12% of these tumours are Hodgkin's disease but do not have data to calculate incidence rates. However, they observed that 80% of their cases presented at an advanced stage, and 52% were of mixed cellularity histology. Findings were similar in two series from New York (Knowles *et al*, 1988; Lowenthal *et al*, 1988) and one from Spain (Serrano *et al*, 1990). Frequent opportunistic infections and poor clinical response were common to all these reports. Thus although the effect on

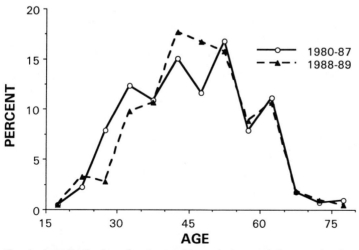

Fig. 1. Age distribution of patients with cervical cancer diagnosed at the Department of Pathology of the University Teaching Hospital, Lusaka, Zambia, 1980–1989 (from Elem B and Patil P, unpublished data, published with permission)

Hodgkin's disease incidence is uncertain, HIV infection has been consistently associated with increased aggressiveness of the disease.

Considered together, cancer registry analyses have failed to detect large increases in cancers overall or of particular types other than non-Hodgkin lymphoma or Kaposi's sarcoma. Associations with the incidence of Hodgkin's disease, anal carcinoma and hepatoma have been present inconsistently and further scrutiny of these data will be necessary, the effect on Hodgkin's disease outcome notwithstanding. Furthermore, the data from these registries apply only for 1987–1988 and thus do not reflect the potential impact of therapy, which has substantially prolonged survival and decreased the incidence of life threatening AIDS defining illnesses. Thus, as was observed in congenital immunodeficiency states, the pattern of tumour occurrence may change as longer latency tumours arise following prolonged survival with sustained immunodeficiency. Already, Pluda *et al* (1990) have documented in a small series a striking excess of lymphomas in severely immunocompromised long-term survivors of HIV infection.

Cohort Studies

The most direct method of identifying HIV-cancer associations is by studies of populations infected with HIV. The National Cancer Institute has been following the appearance of HIV in subjects with haemophilia since the early 1980s (Goedert *et al*, 1989). There are 17 participating treatment centres following 1770 subjects, including 1067 who are HIV positive. Cancers developing in members of this cohort have been monitored. Apart from non-Hodgkin lymphoma and Kaposi's sarcoma, there has been no excess of cancers in this population: 8.0 cases observed versus 8.3 expected (Rabkin CS and Goedert JJ, unpublished observation).

An important distinction between non-Hodgkin lymphoma and Kaposi's sarcoma is the extent of immunosuppression preceding diagnosis: non-Hodgkin lymphoma occurs almost exclusively in severely immunodepressed individuals, whereas Kaposi's sarcoma may occur at any time. In our prospective cohort study of homosexual men, Kaposi's sarcoma occurred at a constant rate of about 2.4% per year between 3 and 8 years after seroconversion, whereas the rate of non-Hodgkin lymphoma increased from 0.8% to 2.6% during this period (Fig. 2; Rabkin and Goedert, 1990).

We have examined the risk of anal epithelial abnormalities (atypia and dysplasia) in this cohort. HIV infection was associated with both increased prevalence and quantity of human papilloma virus (HPV) in anal samples, including HPV types 16/18, which have been linked to carcinoma of the cervix (Caussy *et al*, 1990).

Anal epithelial abnormalities were more frequent in men with both HIV and HPV than in those with either virus alone. Immunodeficiency, as measured by CD4+ T lymphocyte counts, has also been associated with the presence of HPV in HIV infected men (Melbye *et al*, 1990). In a study of more severely immunosuppressed men with AIDS or other serious HIV disease,

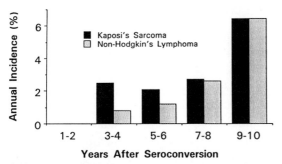

Fig. 2. Annual incidence rates of Kaposi's sarcoma and non-Hodgkin lymphoma by year after seroconversion in 130 HIV infected homosexual men from New York and Washington. By June 1, 1990, Kaposi's sarcoma had developed in 15 subjects and non-Hodgkin lymphoma in 9. (From Rabkin and Goedert, 1990)

15% had anal epithelial neoplasia and 2% had carcinoma in situ (Palefsky *et al*, 1990). However, the importance of these lesions as precursors to anal cancer is unproven.

Similarly, women with HIV infection are at greater risk of cervical HPV infection and cervical intraepithelial neoplasia. In a study of 67 women, 17 of 35 (49%) HIV positive women and 8 of 32 (25%) HIV negative women had HPV detectable by Southern blot (Feingold *et al*, 1990). Eleven of 22 (50%) seropositive women with HIV related symptoms had squamous epithelial lesions on cervical cytology, compared with 3 of 13 (23%) symptom free HIV positive women and only 3 of 32 (9%) HIV negative women. In another cohort, immunosuppression, as measured by CD4+ T lymphocyte count and lymphocyte functional assays, was associated with cervical dysplasia and neoplasia, including invasive carcinoma (Schafer *et al*, 1990).

Other cohorts of HIV infected individuals are still being followed for cancer incidence. However, these studies all include few individuals, and when analyzed individually, they may have insufficient power to detect less common cancer associations.

Case-control Studies

Another way to detect associations between HIV and cancer is by case-control studies. The Atlanta Tumor Registry has lately reported their findings in 44 cases of Hodgkin's disease. Seven of 12 (58%) Hodgkin's disease cases of mixed cellularity histology proved HIV seropositive, compared with none of 32 cases of other histological classifications, supporting the observations of the earlier case series (Liff *et al*, 1990). Another series from France found that 4 of 51 (8%) Hodgkin's disease cases were HIV seropositive, although seroprevalence rates in the general population were not reported (Devars du Mayne *et al*, 1988).

CONCLUSIONS

We can summarize the evidence for specific malignant diseases as follows. HIV infection is probably associated with a relative increase of mixed cellularity Hodgkin's disease but as yet has not been shown to increase total Hodgkin's disease incidence. Hodgkin's disease in the presence of HIV infection tends to be more advanced at presentation and have a more aggressive clinical course. Cervical and anal neoplasia, which probably have similar aetiologies, seem to be increased in the presence of HIV infection and are accelerated in the presence of consequent immunodeficiency. No increases in cancers at these sites have been substantiated so far, but the long incubation of these tumours may allow HIV related increases to be seen in the future. Squamous cell carcinoma of the skin has been associated with other forms of immunodeficiency and may prove to be related to HIV infection, but so far it has not increased. Malignant melanoma also bears monitoring in relation to immunodeficiency, especially in individuals with dysplastic naevi (Greene *et al*, 1981). There is little evidence that other cancers are increased in the presence of HIV infection. However, cancer registry information may be difficult to interpret because of the lack of data about HIV infection in various cancers. Current cohort studies of HIV infection are all of insufficient size to rule out small but clinically important excesses of other tumours.

In conclusion, the model of immune surveillance as an important mechanism for the prevention of cancers of all types is not borne out in observations of HIV infected subjects. The most tantalizing evidence for HIV associations is found mainly in tumours in which other viral factors appear to be important. This phenomenon is common to the cancer types seen in other forms of immunodeficiency. Surveillance of cancers will continue to provide new information as individuals with HIV infection are observed for a longer period. Advances in treatment for HIV infection will delay further the progression to AIDS and may lead to the appearance of HIV associated cancers that otherwise would not have arisen. Prospective cohort studies will need to be of sufficient size to detect less common cancer associations. Case-control studies of cancers of particular types as well as smaller cohort studies to investigate precancerous lesions will be helpful in the investigation of mechanisms by which HIV may facilitate the appearance of cancer. The presence of immunosuppression due to HIV complicates the treatment of cancers irrespective of its role in producing these cancers and may contribute to a poor prognosis.

SUMMARY

In populations with non-HIV immunodeficiency, non-Hodgkin lymphoma and soft tissue sarcoma, especially Kaposi's sarcoma, are the most prominent tumours, but Hodgkin's disease, gastric carcinoma, squamous cell skin cancer, malignant melanoma, hepatoma, myeloid leukaemia and/or colorectal carcinoma have been linked in various studies. Population based cancer registries and cohort studies of HIV infected persons have generally failed to detect HIV related increases in total cancer incidence or in specific tumours other than non-Hodgkin lymphoma and Kaposi's sarcoma; however, associations with anal carcinoma, hepatoma and Hodgkin's disease have been suggested by some studies. Although not indicating increased risk, HIV induced immunosuppression has been linked to an acceleration of cervical and anal neoplasia and to increased aggressiveness of Hodgkin's disease with a relative excess of the mixed cellularity type. Advances in treatment for HIV infection will delay progression to AIDS and may allow an altered natural history to emerge, including the occurrence of excesses of additional cancer types.

References

Bacchetti P and Moss AR (1989) Incubation period of AIDS in San Francisco. *Nature* **338** 251–253

Beral V, Peterman TA, Berkelman RL and Jaffe HW (1990) Kaposi's sarcoma among persons with AIDS: a sexually transmitted infection? *Lancet* **335** 123–128

Biggar RJ, Horm J, Lubin JH, Goedert JJ, Greene MH and Fraumeni JF (1985) Cancer trends in a population at risk of acquired immunodeficiency syndrome. *Journal of the National Cancer Institute* **74** 793–797

Biggar RJ, Burnett W, Mikl J and Nasca P (1989) Cancer among New York men at risk of acquired immunodeficiency syndrome. *International Journal of Cancer* **43** 979–985

Blohme I and Brynger H (1985) Malignant disease in renal transplant patients. *Transplantation* **39** 23–25

Caussy D, Goedert JJ, Palefsky J *et al* (1990). Interaction of human immunodeficiency and papilloma viruses: association with anal epithelial abnormality in homosexual men. *International Journal of Cancer* **46** 214–219

Devars du Mayne JF, Teillet-Thiebaud F, Pulick M and Courton F (1988) Seropositivity to HIV in Hodgkin's disease. *Lancet* **ii** 1024

Feingold Vermund SH, Burk RD, Kelley KF *et al* (1990) Cervical cytologic abnormalities and papillomavirus in women infected with human immunodeficiency virus. *Journal of Acquired Immune Deficiency Syndrome* **3** 896–903

Filipovich AH, Spector BD and Kersey J (1980) Immunodeficiency in humans as a risk factor in the development of malignancy. *Preventive Medicine* **9** 252–259

Goedert JJ, Kessler CM, Aledort LM *et al* (1989) A prospective study of human immunodeficiency virus type 1 infection and the development of AIDS in subjects with hemophilia. *New England Journal of Medicine* **321** 1141–1148

Greene MH, Young TI and Clark WH (1981) Malignant melanoma in renal transplant recipients. *Lancet* **i** 1196–1199

Harnly ME, Swan SH and Kelter A (1989) Reply to Re: Temporal trends in the incidence of non-Hodgkin's lymphoma and selected malignancies in a population with high incidence of acquired immunodeficiency syndrome (AIDS). *American Journal of Epidemiology* **130** 1069–1071

Harwood AR, Osoba D, Hofsteder SL *et al* (1979) Kaposi's sarcoma in recipients of renal transplants. *American Journal of Medicine* **67** 759–765

Hoover RH and Fraumeni JF (1973) Risk of cancer in renal-transplant recipients. *Lancet* **ii** 55–57

Kaplan MH, Susin M, Pahwa SG *et al* (1987) Neoplastic complications of HTLV-III infection: lymphomas and solid tumors. *American Journal of Medicine* **82** 389–396

Kersey JH, Shapiro RS and Filipovich AH (1988) Relationship of immunodeficiency to lymphoid malignancy. *Pediatric Infectious Disease Journal* **7** S10–S12

Kinlen LJ, Sheil AGR, Peto J and Doll R (1979) Collaborative United Kingdom-Australasian study of cancer in patients treated with immunosuppressive drugs. *British Medical Journal* **2** 1461–1466

Knowles DM, Chamulak GA, Subar M *et al* (1988) Lymphoid neoplasia associated with the acquired immunodeficiency syndrome (AIDS): the New York University Medical Center experience with 105 patients (1981–1986). *Annals of Internal Medicine* **108** 744–753

Liff JM, Eley JW, Khabbaz RF, Selik RM and Chan WC (1990) HIV seropositivity and Hodgkin's lymphoma. *Abstracts of the 30th Interscience Conference on Antimicrobial Agents and Chemotherapy,* Atlanta, Georgia, October 21–24. Abstract **1121** p. 273

Lowenthal DA, Straus DJ, Campbell SW, Gold JWM, Clarkson BS and Koziner B (1988) AIDS-related lymphoid neoplasia: the Memorial Hospital experience. *Cancer* **61** 2325–2337

Melbye M, Palefsky J, Gonzales J, Ryder L and Biggar RJ (1990) Immune status as a determinant of human papillomavirus detection and its correlation with anal epithelial abnormalities. *International Journal of Cancer* **46** 203–206

Monfardini S, Vaccher E, Lazzarin A *et al* (1990) Characterization of AIDS-associated tumors in Italy: report of 435 cases of an IVDA-based series. *Cancer Detection and Prevention* **14** 391–393

Mott MG (1984) Childhood non-Hodgkin's lymphoma. *Cancer Surveys* **3** 673–690

Ourcy WL and Jakubek DJ (1987) Multiple squamous cell carcinomas and human immunodeficiency virus infection. *Annals of Internal Medicine* **106** 334

Palefsky JM, Gonzales J, Greenblatt RM, Ahn DK and Hollander H (1990) Anal intraepithelial neoplasia and anal papillomavirus infection among homosexual males with group IV HIV disease. *Journal of the American Medical Association* **263** 2911–2916

Pluda JM, Yarchoan R, Jaffe ES *et al* (1990) Development of opportunistic non-Hodgkin's lymphoma in a cohort of patients with severe HIV infection on long-term antiretroviral therapy. *Annals of Internal Medicine* **113** 276–282

Purtilo DJ and Linder J (1983) Oncological consequences of impaired immune surveillance against ubiquitous viruses. *Journal of Clinical Immunology* **3** 197–206

Rabkin CS and Goedert JJ (1990) Risk of non-Hodgkin lymphoma and Kaposi's sarcoma in homosexual men. *Lancet* **336** 248–249

Rabkin CS, Biggar RJ and Horm JW (1991) Increasing incidence of cancers associated with the human immunodeficiency virus epidemic. *International Journal of Cancer* **43** 692–696

Robert NJ and Schneiderman H (1984) Hodgkin's disease and the acquired immunodeficiency syndrome. *Annals of Internal Medicine* **101** 142–143

Schafer A, Friedmann W, Mielke M, Schwartlander B and Koch MA (1990) Increased frequency of cervical dysplasia/neoplasia in HIV-infected women is related to the extent of immunosuppression. *Final Program and Abstracts of the Sixth International Conference on AIDS* **3** 215

Serrano M, Bellas C, Campo E *et al* (1990) Hodgkin's disease in patients with antibodies to human immunodeficiency virus: a study of 22 patients. *Cancer* **65** 2248–2254

Tirelli U, Vaccher E, Rezza G *et al* (1989) Hodgkin's disease in association with acquired immunodeficiency syndrome (AIDS): a report on 36 patients. *Acta Oncologica* **28** 637–639

Winkelstein W, Lyman DM, Padian NS *et al* (1987) Sexual practices and the risk of infection by the human immunodeficiency virus: The San Francisco Men's Health Study. *Journal of the American Medical Association* **257** 321–325

The authors are responsible for the accuracy of the references.

Biographical Notes

Anne Bayley qualified from Cambridge University and the Middlesex Hospital Medical School in 1958. She worked in rural Northern Rhodesia for two years before training in general surgery in Britain and joined the Ghana Medical School in 1968. In 1971 she went as lecturer to the University Teaching Hospital in Zambia, ending her stay as Professor of Surgery in 1990. She was head of the department in Lusaka from 1980 to 1986, a member of the council of the Association of Surgeons of East Africa from 1977 to 1989 and chairman of the Association in 1983. During the 1970s she was interested in hepatocellular carcinoma and hepatitis B infection. Since 1983 she has studied HIV related Kaposi's sarcoma and the effects of AIDS on families and society in Africa.

Valerie Beral is the Director of the Imperial Cancer Research Fund's Cancer Epidemiology Unit. A graduate of Sydney, Australia, her introduction to epidemiology was as a medical student assisting in a health survey of New Guinea highlanders. After some years of clinical practice, she joined the staff of the Epidemiology Department of the London School of Hygiene and Tropical Medicine. She has a longstanding interest in the aetiology of cancer in women, including the role of sexually transmitted infections in cervical cancer. During a sabbatical year at the Centers for Disease Control in Atlanta, Georgia, she had the opportunity of expanding her work on transmissible agents in cancer by collaborating in studies of the epidemiology of Kaposi's sarcoma and other HIV associated cancers.

William A Blattner is Chief, Viral Epidemiology Section, National Cancer Institute, Bethesda, Maryland. He graduated from Washington University in St Louis, Missouri, with subsequent training at the University of Rochester, Cornell University and in the medical oncology training program of the National Cancer Institute. Prior to his current research focus on human retroviruses, he studied the aetiology of cancer in high risk families, especially immunological and immunogenetic aspects. This background has been relevant to his work in studies of both the human T lymphotrophic and the human immunodeficiency viruses and their relationship to cancer. He is Co-Editor-in-Chief of the *Journal of AIDS*.

Aby Buchbinder graduated in medicine at McGill University, Montreal, and later trained at the National Cancer Insitute. He is presently Research Assistant Professor at New York University Medical Center and runs his retrovirology laboratory at the Manhattan Veterans' Affairs Medical Center.

Clay J Cockerell, MD, is Assistant Professor of Dermatology and Pathology at the University of Texas Southwestern Medical School in Dallas, Texas. His undergraduate medical training was at Baylor College of Medicine and postgraduate medical education was at New York University Medical Center, New York. Dr Cockerell has written extensively on cutaneous manifestations of human immunodeficiency virus infection and was instrumental in recognizing the newly described condition, bacillary epithelioid angiomatosis. As a diagnostic dermatopathologist, he has had extensive experience with the histopathological features of Kaposi's sarcoma, both the classical and the AIDS related types.

Dorothy H Crawford qualified in medicine from St Thomas's Hospital Medical School, London, in 1968, and then trained in pathology. She gained her PhD from Bristol University in 1976 while studying in the Department of Pathology, headed by Professor MA Epstein. She held research assistant appointments in the Department of Immunology, Royal Free Hospital, and the Department of Haematology, University College, London, before moving to the Royal Postgraduate Medical School as Senior Lecturer and later Reader in Virology. She has recently been appointed Professor of Microbiology at the London School of Hygiene and Tropical Medicine, where she heads a group working on the cellular and molecular aspects of Epstein-Barr virus infection.

Alvin E Friedman-Kien, MD, is Professor of Dermatology and Microbiology and Director of the Immunovirology Laboratory, Center for AIDS Research, New York University Medical Center. He was the first investigator to bring to light epidemic Kaposi's sarcoma and is currently interested in the aetiology and pathophysiology of Kaposi's sarcoma.

Seymour Grufferman received his MD from the State University of New York, Syracuse, in 1964, trained in paediatrics and received his PhD in epidemiology from the Harvard School of Hygiene and Public Health in 1979. He is Professor and Chairman, Department of Clinical Epidemiology and Preventive Medicine, University of Pittsburgh School of Medicine.

Brian G Herndier obtained a PhD in chemistry at the California Institute of Technology in 1981 after undergraduate training at the University of British Columbia. After completion of an MD in 1983 he went to Stanford for residency training in pathology, including an immunodiagnosis fellowship under Roger Warnke and Ronald Dorfman. After completion of laboratory medicine residency at the University of California at San Francisco, he became an Assistant Professor in Residence in Pathology and Laboratory Medicine at UCSF, based at the San Francisco General Hospital. Current research interests have focused on the pathogenesis of AIDS and HIV lymphomas.

Harold W Jaffe, MD, received his undergraduate degree in genetics from the University of California at Berkeley and his medical degree from the University of California at Los Angeles. He trained in internal medicine and infectious diseases at UCLA Hospital and the University of Chicago Hospital. Since 1981, he has been one of a group of investigators studying the epidemiology of AIDS at the Centers for Disease Control in Atlanta. During the 1989–1990 academic year, he was a Visiting Professor at the Institute of Cancer Research in London.

Lawrence D Kaplan, MD, is an Assistant Clinical Professor of Medicine in the AIDS/Oncology Division at San Francisco General Hospital. He received his medical training at the Center for the Health Sciences, University of California at Los Angeles, and at the Boston City Hospital. He conducts basic and clinical research in the biology, diagnosis and therapy of HIV related malignancies. His particular area of interest is HIV related lymphoma.

Jenny Luxton graduated from Kings College, London University, in 1987, where she studied microbiology. She worked for three years as a research assistant in the Department of Virology, Royal Postgraduate Medical School, before moving to the London School of Hygiene and Tropical Medicine. She is currently working for a PhD, studying T cell immune responses to Epstein-Barr virus infected cells in normal and immunosuppressed individuals.

Donald W Northfelt, MD, is a research fellow in the AIDS/Oncology Division at San Francisco General Hospital. He received his medical training at the University of Minnesota School of Medicine in Minneapolis and at the Center for the Health Sciences, University of California at Los Angeles. He is currently completing a fellowship in haematology and oncology at the University of California at San Francisco. He conducts clinical research in the diagnosis and treatment of HIV related malignancies, haematological disorders and opportunistic infections.

Gunta Iris Obrams received her MD from Albany Medical College in 1977, trained in preventive medicine and received her PhD in epidemiology from Johns Hopkins University in 1988. She is Chief of the Extramural Programs Branch, Epidemiology and Biostatistic Program, National Cancer Institute.

Thomas A Peterman, MD, MSc, is Chief of the Viral Studies Section, Division of STD/HIV Prevention, at the Centers for Disease Control. He received his undergraduate degree from Kalamazoo College, medical degree from the University of Michigan and MSc in epidemiology from the London School of Hygiene and Tropical Medicine. He trained in internal medicine at the Ohio State University Hospitals. He has studied the epidemiology of transfusion associated AIDS and the heterosexual transmission of HIV. He is currently studying the prevention of HIV and other viral sexually transmitted infections.

Charles S Rabkin graduated from the Medical Education Program of Brown University and has an MSc in epidemiology from the London School of Hygiene and Tropical Medicine. He trained in internal medicine at the University of Colorado. His epidemiology training was at the US Centers for Disease Control, and through that he was assigned to the New York City AIDS Program from 1984 to 1986 and the Hospital Infections Program from 1986 to 1987. He is currently the HIV-Cancer Coordinator for the Viral Epidemiology Section, National Cancer Institute. His research interests include non-Hodgkin lymphoma and Kaposi's sarcoma as well as other HIV-cancer associations.

J Alero Thomas qualified in medicine from St Mary's Hospital Medical School, London, in 1970. After various house appointments both in Britain and Nigeria, she won a Commonwealth Scholarship to Somerville College, Oxford, to carry out research into red cell metabolism, which led to an MSc thesis. She held research assistant posts in the Department of Immunology, Royal Free Hospital (1978–1981), and the Department of Histopathology, Royal Marsden Hospital (1978–1984), before being appointed a non-clinical research scientist at the Imperial Cancer Research Fund, London, where she runs the Histopathology Unit. Her research interests include an immunohistological approach to the study of B and T cell ontogeny and Epstein-Barr virus associated lesions in immunocompromised patients.

Robin A Weiss, PhD, HonMRCP, FRCPath, is Director of Research and Professor of Viral Oncology at the Chester Beatty Laboratories, Institute of Cancer Research, London. He received his undergraduate and research training in zoology at University College London and has worked in the USA, Czechoslovakia and India. From 1980 to 1989 he was Director of the Institute of Cancer Research. He has had a long-term interest in retroviruses.

Index

LIST OF PREVIOUS ISSUES

VOLUME 1 1982

No. 1: Inheritance of Susceptibility to Cancer in Man
Guest Editor: W F Bodmer

No. 2: Maturation and Differentiation in Leukaemias
Guest Editor: M F Greaves

No. 3: Experimental Approaches to Drug Targeting
Guest Editors: A J S Davies and M J Crumpton

No. 4: Cancers Induced by Therapy
Guest Editor: I Penn

VOLUME 2 1983

No. 1: Embryonic & Germ Cell Tumours in Man and Animals
Guest Editor: R L Gardner

No. 2: Retinoids and Cancer
Guest Editor: M B Sporn

No. 3: Precancer
Guest Editor: J J DeCosse

No. 4: Tumour Promotion and Human Cancer
Guest Editors: T J Slaga and R Montesano

VOLUME 3 1984

No. 1: Viruses in Human and Animal Cancers
Guest Editors: J Wyke and R Weiss

No. 2: Gene Regulation in the Expression of Malignancy
Guest Editor: L Sachs

No. 3: Consistent Chromosomal Aberrations and Oncogenes in Human Tumours
Guest Editor: J D Rowley

No. 4: Clinical Management of Solid Tumours in Childhood
Guest Editor: T J McElwain

VOLUME 4 1985

No. 1: Tumour Antigens in Experimental and Human Systems
Guest Editor: L W Law

No. 2: Recent Advances in the Treatment and Research in Lymphoma and Hodgkin's Disease
Guest Editor: R Hoppe

No. 3: Carcinogenesis and DNA Repair
Guest Editor: T Lindahl

No. 4: Growth Factors and Malignancy
Guest Editors: A B Roberts and M B Sporn

VOLUME 5 1986

No. 1: Drug Resistance
Guest Editors: G Stark and H Calvert

No. 2: Biochemical Mechanisms of Oncogene Activity: Proteins Encoded by Oncogenes
Guest Editors: H E Varmus and J M Bishop

No. 3: Hormones and Cancer: 90 Years after Beatson
Guest Editor: R D Bulbrook

No. 4: Experimental, Epidemiological and Clinical Aspects of Liver Carcinogenesis
Guest Editor: E Farber

VOLUME 6 1987

No. 1: Naturally Occurring Tumours in Animals as a Model for Human Disease
Guest Editors: D Onions and W Jarrett

No. 2: New Approaches to Tumour Localization
Guest Editor: K Britton

No. 3: Psychological Aspects of Cancer
Guest Editor: S Greer

No. 4: Diet and Cancer
Guest Editors: C Campbell and L Kinlen

VOLUME 7 1988

No. 1: Pain and Cancer
Guest Editor: G W Hanks